Bridging *the* Gap to Oneness

Dr. Barbara's Integrative Guide To Healing & Wholeness

Dr. Barbara Gordon-Cohen, D.O.

WHAT PEOPLE ARE SAYING

"Bridging the Gap to Oneness is a personal account of healing and transformation from skilled Dr. Barbara Gordon-Cohen, D.O. Dr. Barbara explains in her story-telling style how emotional healing and life-style changes can lead to better health and cures to illness. She talks honestly about her own journey, her patients, and the experiences that led her to a deep understanding of the mind-body-emotion-spirit connection and the true causes of illness. She gives us hope that we can change, heal, and cure through many practices from eastern/western medicine to food to dance! I've had the pleasure to dance with Dr. Barbara and experience her shining light in person. What a gift!"

~ Toni Bergins
M.ED. Founder of JourneyDance™,
a transformational movement practice
www.journeydance.com

"Dr Barbara takes us on a personal journey of discovery, realization and healing. She teaches that any health issue needs to be treated holistically and that symptoms are signs that point us to the underlying causes of our physical and emotional challenges. She demonstrates that there is more than one pathway to healing and, importantly, that when we take the time to stop and really listen to our bodies we are naturally guided to deep healing wisdom. Her book is packed full of inspirational real life stories, practical tips and great healing advice."

~ Brandon Bays
Cellular Healing Authority and
International Bestselling Author of *The Journey*^{TM}
www.thejourney.com

~ ~ ~ ~ ~ ~ ~ ~ ~ ~ ~ ~ ~ ~ ~ ~ ~

"Barbara Gordon-Cohen,D.O. after being a complete physician from the original holistic and alternative medical profession of Osteopathy for 26 years, has contributed to the vernacular this wonderful informative guide to getting answers to complex and everyday medical conditions. Kudos for trying to help the patients who hunger for peace in body, mind and Spirit."

~ Dr. Paul Capobianco, D.O.

"Dr. Barbara Gordon-Cohen, D. O. has written a very readable and highly personal and practical book on how to achieve one's potential. As she describes her own quest for good health, she manages to summarize how various disciplines, such as nutrition and nutritional supplements, osteopathy, acupuncture, homeopathy, yoga, exercise, spiritual fulfillment and many others can be used to achieve wholeness and health in this very stressful and often toxic world. I highly recommend it."

~ Michael B. Schachter, M.D.

Certified Nutrition Specialist (CNS); Board Certified Psychiatrist; Former President of the American College for Advancement in Medicine (ACAM): Owner and Director of the Schachter Center for Complementary Medicine in Suffern NY since 1974.
www.schachtercenter.com

~ ~ ~ ~ ~ ~ ~ ~ ~ ~ ~ ~ ~ ~ ~ ~

"A portrait of holistic healing and the tools to explore for your own journey!"

~ Kelly Brogan, M.D.
Author, *A Mind of Your Own*

Dr. Barbara teaches us about good health by sharing her own personal journey towards mental, emotional, and physical well-being. In addition she shares insights from a number of health modalities including osteopathy, Ayurvedic, acupuncture, yoga, bio identical hormones, and nutrition.

Her book is also significant for repeatedly emphasizing the mind-body connection. Not only in her reference to the work of Dr. John Sarno, but also in relation to her health journey and those of many of her patients. For these reasons I encourage you to read the book as there should be something important for nearly everyone in this book.

~ **David Schechter, M.D.**
Author, *Think Away Your Pain*
and the *Mind-Body Workbook*
Private practice, Culver City, California

ACKNOWLEDGMENTS

I would like to thank my mother, Adele, may she rest in peace, my husband, my children and my father for giving me the support to pursue medicine, the encouragement in pursuing my passions and the space to write this book.

I also have deep gratitude for my editor Miriam Zernis who entered my life at just the right time. I had asked her husband Walter Zernis "out of the blue" while he was in my office as a vitamin representative, if he knew of any editors. He looked at me squarely in the eye and told me, "my wife." The rest is history. I would like to thank Gloria Owens for her keen eye, designing the book cover and interior pages and for her endless patience. My sister for assisting me with the production of the book and writing the chapter on acupuncture. Chrissy Gruninger for being the social media expert and helping bring this book to fruition.

Lastly, I would like to dedicate this book to Patricia Steinley-Davis who was my original writer and editor years ago when I had the initial idea to write this book. She was a wonderful patient of mine who extended herself with her amazing writing skills to get me started on this project. Soon after I moved to Israel, she had passed away suddenly and unexpectedly. I was then sparked to continue the book on her behalf. I know she was my guiding light during this process.

FOREWORD

Dr. Barbara has been a dear and close friend of mine, more like a soulmate since we met over 25 years ago. We were neighbors and clicked right away, having similar backgrounds and interests. We were busy living our lives unconsciously going through our routines of working, having children and raising a family.

We are both in healing professions – myself as a Holistic Midwife/OB/GYN Nurse Practitioner and Dr. Barbara as an Osteopath/Integrative Physician – and we were taking care of everyone else but ourselves. We awoke gradually, and began to journey together into consciousness by traveling to Costa Rica, the Caribbean and Kripalu Center in MA, for R&R, yoga, massage, and breathwork retreats and workshops.

We needed to take breaks from the intensity of our lives, exploring, living fully, laughing, being ourselves, and healing. We fell apart together and literally helped each other through our processes. We have been there for each other in tough times and great times and our healing continues together no matter where we are.

Dr. Barbara inspired my own journey with nutrition, supplements, acupuncture, homeopathy, yoga, breath work, meditation and osteopathic cranial sessions. Dr. Barbara introduced me to Dr. Sarno's method for healing pain, Imago therapy, biofeedback and The Journey™ work. In this process I was able to develop into the integrative holistic nurse midwife and healing practitioner I am today: balanced, empowered and liberated. Today I help thousands of women and their families around the world along their journeys to giving birth, teaching yoga for pregnancy, birth, and postpartum, as well as guiding Clarity Breathwork sessions to help people release past traumas, emotional pain and inner stress.

I knew of Dr. Barbara's healing gifts and magic hands early in our relationship. My daughter, who had chronic ear infections, did not respond to natural remedies that usually worked. It was affecting her ability to hear and learn. I took her to a renowned ENT specialist at a prestigious NYC hospital. He was concerned about the amount of fluid in both her middle ears and recommended surgical tubes right away, to drain the fluid, prevent infection and impairment of her hearing. The doctor reluctantly agreed, to give me four weeks, before doing the surgery. He prescribed another month of high dose antibiotics.

During this time Dr. Barbara treated my daughter with cranial osteopathic manipulation. When I returned to the ENT, he was flabbergasted: the fluid was gone. He told me how impressed he was with the antibiotic regimen. I told him I did not give her the antibiotics. He didn't believe that the osteopathic treatments worked. I did not need his belief. I had my own proof and was so grateful surgery was avoided.

Our vacations together became necessities. We took off from our hectic work schedules, as we planned, coveted & guarded them with care. Ahhhh.... the taste of freedom, joy, fun and play; recharging and restoring, the warm sun and beauty of the tropical Caribbean. The first days of one of our retreats on the beach we played volleyball with the locals and I collided with a man. I heard a crack and felt sudden excruciating pain in my leg. I collapsed to the ground and mourned the ruin of our much needed vacation. Dr. Barbara assessed the situation and treated me osteopathically. I felt an enormous shift & was back to myself the next day. I am one of many of Dr. Barbara's success stories.

I highly recommend Dr. Barbara's book presenting clinical cases treated with integrative modalities, resulting in complete healing for many. "Bridging the Gap to Oneness" intertwines her personal stories of healing, wisdom and intuition. The book is an informative guide to help you on your journey to body-mind-spirit integration and wholeness.

A must read!

~ **Anne Margolis CNM, MSN,**
Certified Yoga Teacher and Clarity Breathwork Practitioner;
Bestselling Author of two books: *Natural Birth Secrets: An Insiders Guide How To Give Birth Holistically, Healthfully and Safely, and Love the Experience*, and *Trauma Release Formula: The Revolutionary Step by Step Program for Eliminating Effects of Childhood Abuse, Trauma, Emotional Pain and Crippling Inner Stress, to Living in Joy without Drugs or Therapy*
www.homesweethomebirth.com

CONTENTS

Bridging *the* Gap to Oneness

Dr. Barbara's Integrative Guide To Healing & Wholeness

Dr. Barbara Gordon-Cohen, D.O.

PART ONE

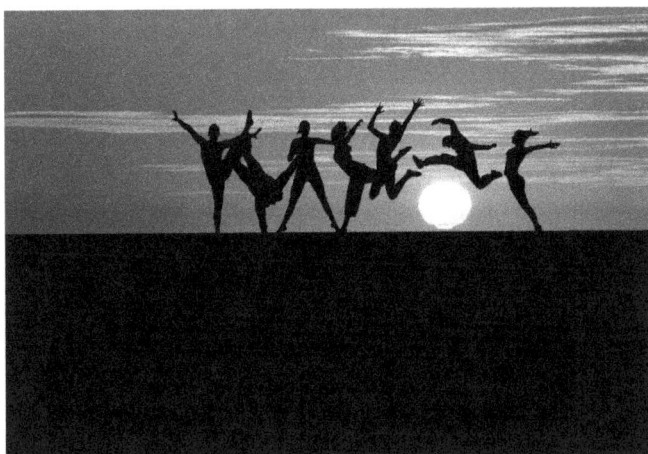

CHAPTER 1

INTRODUCTION INTO OSTEOPATHY

Five-year-old Stevie was brought to my office with a history of chronic sinus infections. He had been on numerous antibiotics, but they were not helping. Upon evaluation, I found he had a high palate that did not allow enough room for his sinuses to drain. This condition can be treated by freeing the bones in the cranium, sacrum, and palate. After five osteopathic cranial treatments, Stevie no longer had any infection. I continued to treat him once a month over a six-month period, and he achieved full recovery – no more sinus infections.

From about the age of 13, I was determined to become a doctor. There were many reasons for the obsession that turned me into a homework machine. I had been a gymnast from the age of five and became very interested in the mechanics of the human body. My mother was an administrator in the manipulative medicine department at an osteopathic medical school, where I could sit in on labs from a young age.

In gymnastics competitions, one is always striving for that "perfect 10" and because of this, it is easy to see why I became a perfectionist in the sport, as well as in my life. Everything went according to my plan – up to a point. I received a gymnastics scholarship, went off to college, trained and studied several hours a day, eating only half portions at meals.

Though no one, not even my coach, asked me to shed pounds, I got my weight down to precisely 105. That was an ideal weight for a gymnast, so I did it because I had seen that a model in a magazine weighed exactly that amount. It was fortunate that 105 was the perfect number because that obsession kept me from developing full-blown anorexia.

It was not enough to just focus on getting a minimum of a B grade on my pre-med courses and getting into medical school: I had to compete on the gymnastics team, study hard and socialize, as well be popular in college.

By the middle of my first semester at college, my "well-rounded" student life was already falling apart. I came down with mononucleosis, showing all the standard symptoms: sore throat, swollen glands and an overwhelming sense of fatigue.

Even though I did not have the stamina to finish a gymnastics routine, my coach pressured me to compete, warning me that I would be a failure in life if I did not stick it out and even worse, I would lose my scholarship. After all, I was under a doctor's care, and the numbers on my blood count were not high enough to justify a medical release from my commitment to the team.

Even back then I realized that I was not being treated as a whole person, just as a set of numbers that did not reflect that I had been half-starving myself, that I needed more sleep than I was getting, that I was doing my team no good and that I was too tired to study properly. The truth was all of this was stressing me to the breaking point.

Norma came to me with IBS (irritable bowel syndrome), complaining of diarrhea and cramping. Focusing on taking a thorough history, I discovered that she drank at least eight glasses of cola every day. Once I knew that her treatment became very simple. Gradually she weaned herself off cola. When Norma stopped drinking soda, she no longer had IBS. Sounds very easy but an allopathic doctor probably would never have discovered the cause of her illness because, typically, the history is no more than a

> *form the patient fills out and most of the time they do not ask about soda usage.*

Somehow, I toughed out my first semester, but in doing so I used up all my physical and emotional resources. Over winter break, I slept 17 hours a day, every day. Stress had sucked all the joy out of 14 years of gymnastics training and performing. When I returned to school, I never felt the same about the sport again.

Toward the end of my second year, I finally decided I had to let gymnastics go and try to get some balance back into my life. This balance is something I still work on until this day. When I told the gymnastics coach my decision, after telling me I would be a quitter in life, she then did a 360 degree turn around and waited until the end of the semester to try to get my scholarship back.

She begged me to let go of my scholarship for someone else. The pressure from her was all about her status and not my personal welfare and illness. In the medical books if an athlete has mononucleosis he or she is not allowed to exercise for a minimum of 6 weeks due to spleen or liver enlargement and possible rupture.

After quitting gymnastics, I felt empty inside. I had lost a large chunk of my identity. It literally felt like someone I was close to had died and I went through a grieving process. I was depressed for some time after quitting the team.

Once the semester was over I took contemplative walks about 10 miles a day, started jazz dance classes, and swimming. It was clear to me that exercise relieved much of my stress.

Very gradually I found ways to be peaceful and replenish myself emotionally and spiritually, though I did not think about it in those terms for a long time. I no longer felt I had to be so controlled with food and the anorexia mentality slowly melted away.

Now in my 50's, I no longer weigh myself and instead just focus on eating healthy foods. I do not eat gluten (wheat, oat, barley and rye) due to gluten intolerance which I developed after the loss of my mother. Gluten can be inflammatory as it is genetically modified and are bodies see it as foreign.

I have learned so much from my patients about gluten. Many had muscular pain, eczema, joint pain and bowel problems all associated with gluten intolerance. Conventional doctors may miss gluten intolerance or sensitivity when lab tests are normal. There is a lab test for gluten intolerance called gliadin antibody testing, however, some people's antibodies for gluten are normal despite their symptoms. I have patients refrain from eating gluten for 4 weeks to see if there is an improvement in their condition. Often, there is.

Medicine is both an art and science. The body is not black and white. It has three dimensions to it – body, mind, and spirit. We are so complex and as a physician, it is my job to find the root cause of illness or prevent illness through these three dimensions.

My spiritual quest was manifesting after I quit gymnastics and ended a relationship with a vivacious guy. He was funny, charming and smart but he was not interested in commitment and truthfully neither was I. At some point, he said we'd have to end our relationship as he did not want it to lead to marriage. He was the first love of my life and my heart was broken.

The combination of quitting gymnastics and losing my best friend was very traumatic for me. I had to find myself again.

It all hit me hard one day during Yom Kippur. I always felt out of place during this holiday, as there were very few Jews at my school. I did not go to synagogue as I did as a child, instead, I went to the chemistry lab.

After the lab, I started to wheeze and had to go to the student medical clinic to get my breathing checked and back to normal. It is interesting that in acupuncture the lungs and colon are the meridians associated with grief.

Well, I was grieving!

I was not observing this important holiday with my family. I did fast on this day and at the end of the fast, I went to the health food store to buy nuts and raisins. I bumped into a friend who was also breaking her fast. We both sat outside and ate as she told me all about her semester in Israel. I was so intrigued that I told myself in my heart that I had to get there one day, somehow.

My curiosity, my grief, and perhaps being a minority in college had made me start thinking about G-d and the path to take to get closer to G-d. I began my first spiritual search on a ground level by taking a Hebrew course, even though I did not have much time as a pre-med student. I didn't have much of a religious background and had never attended Hebrew school.

There were five students in my class. The teacher was a Rabbi and he taught us Hebrew and showed us films on Israel. I was falling in love with this country and would even take walks thinking about the history of Israel and the beautiful land that I wanted so much to see.

Around the same time, I bought a book on yoga and started doing sun salutations. I found myself on a holistic spiritual quest that sprang, seemingly, from nowhere.

Yet I somehow understood that these feelings were closely tied to my physical and emotional health. I had learned that when I bottled up my emotions, I got sick. In fact, if my behavior became extreme in any way: too much studying, not enough exercise or food or sleep, I would get a sore throat and swollen glands. What were the physical and emotional connections? The physical sensitivity I now know had come from the Epstein Barr Virus due to having had mononucleosis and the emotional side were the stressors that I had put on myself as well as the stressors that were not in my control.

Sara came to my office complaining of numbness in both arms. She was 25 years, single and had been complaining of numbness in both arms for 6 months. She had already been to a neurologist and had undergone nerve conduction studies, labs and a physical. The doctor had declared her fine and that her symptoms were "just in her head", an unhelpful diagnosis in every way.

Aggravated by the neurologist's words and manner, Sara decided to try a different type of doctor, a more integrative physician. As I took her history and asked about her family, I learned that her mother had died of breast cancer when Sara was just a teenager. I asked if she had been close to her mother. "Yes, very close," she said. How had she dealt with her mother's loss, I asked. Sara had said she just kept going. Had she grieved or cried? "No", she said, "I just moved forward."

I explained that her symptoms could have arisen from the fact that she never fully grieved the loss of her mother. I suggested that she go into therapy to process the grief of losing her mother.

Even as I spoke these words Sara started to cry, as if someone had finally pinpointed the center of her pain. Sara did see a therapist. After 2 sessions, her numbness-both physical and mental – was gone.

The process of healing and the losses that occurred in college slowly evolved in an interesting direction for which I was caught off guard. With the encouragement of my parents, I spent six weeks during my winter break with my aunt and uncle who were both artists. They lived near the beach on eastern Long Island. I found walking on the beach very peaceful and healing.

The first thing my Aunt did was take me shopping – not for clothes, but for beads and decorative fabrics. She soon got me interested in decorating T-shirts and barrettes. This simple, creative activity gave me a sense of artistic fulfillment I had never experienced before. I had never taken time from my studies and sports to explore my creative side, and it felt wonderful to indulge it.

I also walked and walked on the beach on those bleak, chilly winter days – up to seven hours at a time, meditating on my identity.

Who was I? What was my purpose? Had I lost part of myself giving up a competitive sport? Had I found a new part of myself designing t-shirts and barrettes?

I also often thought of a video I had seen about Israel. Was my empty feeling physical, mental, emotional, spiritual or all the above? Could filling it be as simple as picking up a shell on the beach, taking a closer look, and deciding either to put it in my pocket or toss it away?

Sheila, a 50-year-old teacher, married with 2 children, came to me in an extremely anxious state, unable to function at her job or within her family. She had already visited her internist, complaining of pain in her right ear. The doctor looked in her ears and although he did not find any infection he gave her antibiotics anyway.

When she returned a week later she showed no sign of improvement. Her doctor then recommended that she see a dentist. The dentist told Sheila that she had TMJ (temporomandibular joint) pain. He made her an upper bite guard to prevent clenching and thus pain. With the guard in place, Sheila's pain only worsened – it spread to her neck and she experienced a lot of anxiety. One night her worried husband, not knowing what else to do, convinced her to go to a psychiatric center nearby. She was given valium and sent home. She came to my office after all this, still without a clue to the source of her pain. Taking her history, I asked if she was driven, a perfectionist or people-pleaser. She admitted she was, and this was verified by what she told me about her family dynamics. She was a constant caretaker of her children, husband, and students. This gave me a clue that the pain might have an emotional component.

Upon examination, I found a trigger point in her right trapezius – a large muscle that stretches from the back of her head and inserts on the shoulder and the midback, (a trigger point is a muscle that, when touched, refers pain to another area.) People who have chronic pain often have trigger points.

I treated Sheila's trigger point with a lidocaine injection, a numbing agent and then proceeded to manually examine her cranial mechanism. The bones of Sheila's cranium did not move – at all.

The cranium is comprised of many different bones with sutures and bevels and grooves that allow for motion of the cranial bones which are surrounding the brain.

Dr. William Sutherland founded Cranial Oste-opathy in the early 1900's by doing experiments on his own and studying the anatomy of the disarticulated skull and what lies beneath. At one point during his experiments, he took 2 baseball gloves and placed one on top of his head and one under his chin and tied them together with shoe-string until his head was compressed tightly. His wife found him in his study hours later "passed out". He had created a cranial compression where no cerebrospinal fluid could move as the bony components of the skull were compressed not al-lowing for fluid fluctuation of the cerebral spinal fluid within the brain. The Cerebrospinal fluid nourishes the brain and spinal cord and is the highest known element in the body. We cannot live without this fluid which drives all other fluids in the body.

Sheila's cranial mechanism was stuck. The dental guard the dentist had made for her upper palate had shut down her cranial mechanism by creating a cranial compression. I util-ized a technique that decompresses the cranium to get the bones moving again. On her follow-up visit, Sheila was a new woman – able to return to work without pain and anxiety.

Of course, her perfectionistic tendency remained, so she needed to remind herself from time to time to ease up on her expectations of herself. I treated Sheila a few more times, advising her to get rid of her mouth guard and take up meditation, yoga or walking to help her relax and prevent future episodes of pain and anxiety. She continued to have good health.

CHAPTER 2

MY CAREER DECISION

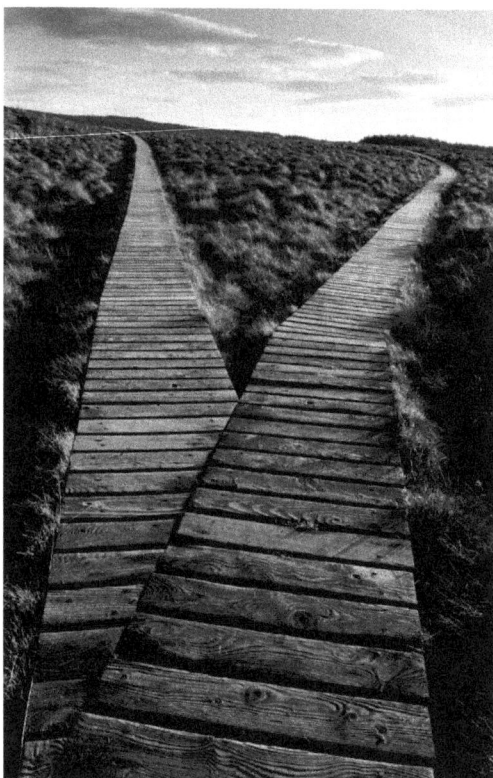

I returned to college wondering if becoming an osteopathic physician was the right choice for me. I was so young – how was I to know?

But as I thought about what I had learned about the body through athletics, I knew I wanted to find out more about physical therapy and chiropractic as well as osteopathy.

During winter break in my fourth year of college, two of my friends who were also trying to make similar decisions decided we would plan a cross country trip and visit osteopathic and chiropractic schools.

Besides really enjoying our trip, we were all on a mutual journey to figure out what we wanted to do one day. One of my friends was in a physical therapy program at my college already and the other one had a father who was a chiropractor, so he was leaning toward chiropractic school. I had my osteopathic mentors from the osteopathic school that my mom worked at, so I was leaning towards osteopathy.

I have to say being twenty and seeing the chiropractic school in Los Angeles almost had me convinced that this would be the route I would take. Why? They had a beautiful swimming pool with diving boards and a gym. That is how a twenty-year-old mind thinks. I was almost convinced.

I made my final decision when I was in Florida where I visited a friend of my parents who was a family practitioner and practiced osteopathy. He pointed out that osteopathic medical training in the United States is far broader than training for chiropractic or physical therapy.

While osteopathy includes the hands-on diagnosis and treatment of the mechanics of the physical body, in which I was so interested, I would also be treating the whole patient and would be learning about all areas of medicine.

Osteopathy was the way for me to keep all my options open. I felt very young to be making such an important life and career decision based on so little life experience but also felt very lucky to have found the information I needed at just the right time and also, to have had role models in the osteopathic profession.

Helen, the mother of a newborn, brought her child to my office. Her lactation consultant had told her the baby was not getting enough milk, so Helen was using a special device that attached to her breast to pump more milk to the baby. I examined the baby osteopathically and felt that the baby had a high palate, which could make nursing more problematic. I also felt that the 2 bones that house the nerves that allow for sucking and swallowing were not moving properly and there was restriction between these bones (the Temporal and Occipital bone). I gave the baby a cranial treatment to restore motion of these bones and to improve the position of the palate. This gentle treatment released restrictions of the nerves involved in sucking and swallowing and after only 2 treatments the baby no longer needed the special nursing device and after three sessions he was feeding well on his own.

CHAPTER 3

THE CHAKRA SYSTEM & ISRAEL

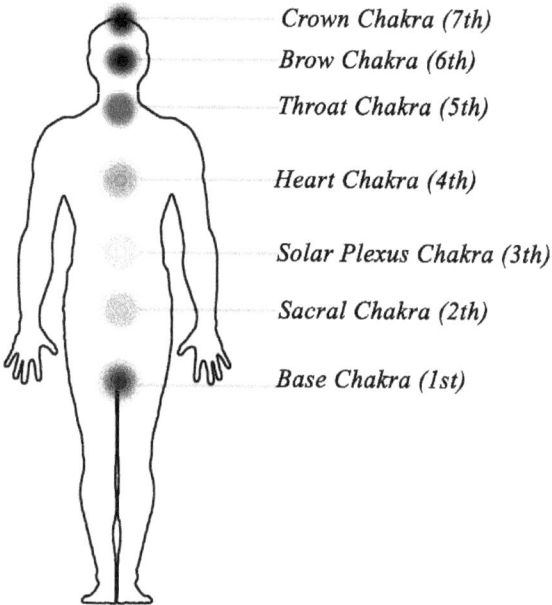

Crown Chakra (7th)
Brow Chakra (6th)
Throat Chakra (5th)

Heart Chakra (4th)

Solar Plexus Chakra (3th)

Sacral Chakra (2th)

Base Chakra (1st)

The last year of college, I had my pre-med finals. Taking the MCATs (medical entrance exams required to get into medical school) turned into a very stressful ordeal.

In my nervousness, I misunderstood the time the second half of the test would begin. During the lunch break, I went off to meditate and relax, and

when I returned, I was 30 minutes late, which totally rattled me. I misinterpreted the time by
twenty minutes and now I was late for reading
comprehension, my weakest area of the test. I just
froze and put in any answer.

Unfortunately, due to the poor score I received on
this part, I had to take the exam again. To prepare
again and wait until the summer until I received
notice from medical schools took a toll on me.

I started to suffer from stomach burning and pain
as I anxiously awaited admission acceptance into
medical school. I finally went to a recommended
gastroenterologist sent me for x-rays of my stomach and all was normal. He then asked me if I was
overly stressed. The minute he asked me this
question I began to sob. All the pent-up anger,
resentment, and fear poured out. Through my
sobs, I explained about having to take MCATs
twice and not liking standardized tests.

At that point, the doctor literally abandoned me.
He turned on his heel and left the consultation
room. I could see him out in the hallway lighting
up a cigarette to soothe his nerves. In the face of
my emotions, he was helpless to do anything but
wait it out; he had nothing to offer. My body,
however, understood perfectly well. After this
huge emotion-purging cry, the pain in my
stomach simply disappeared on its own.

I want to be very clear about the episode. My

stomach hurt, so I went to a doctor who specialized in the digestive system. He examined me, did testing and labs and told me nothing was wrong.

If the doctor had asked if I was stressed, whether he knew it or not, he was on the cusp of solving the mystery. But when he walked out of the room, the message was that a physically healthy person was wasting the doctor's highly specialized time. My own body was wiser than both of us.

First, it signaled to me that something was wrong, and it kept signaling until I paid attention to the feelings and emotions I had bottled up. Once I released my feelings my body's job was done – I had rebalanced myself.

I believe in "the body's inherent wisdom": its physical symptoms can signal an inner imbalance in the physical, emotional or spiritual realm and it is up to us as healers to find out where this imbalance is coming from.

The Chakra system of healing, derived from the Sanskrit (Hindu) word meaning "circle" is described as a spinning wheel of light or energy channels through which the life force (prana) moves.

There are 7 chakras – each relating to a different organ system, emotion and spiritual energy in our bodies. Western practices of using Chakras can be traced back to the 18th century to treat diseases.

The first chakra is connected to the low back and sacrum and how we relate to our physical environment, our tribe or community, and our finances.

The second Chakra is connected to the sex organs, lying below the umbilicus (belly button) and is related to our relationships, sexuality, and communication with our partners.

The third Chakra is in the solar plexus below the sternum, is connected to the digestive organs and is related to our inner power, strength, and confidence.

The fourth Chakra is the heart center connected to our emotions and feelings in the heart area at the sternum.

The fifth chakra is in the area of our throat, is connected to the thyroid, throat, parathyroid glands and is related to our inner voice, speaking up for oneself and using one's speech appropriately.

The sixth chakra is between our eyebrows or 3rd eye point is connected to the pituitary gland, the master gland of the body and is related to our inner wisdom and intellect and the seventh Chakra is at the top or crown of the head, in the brain and above, and relates to our connection to the universe and spirit.

Each chakra has a different color and sound and

relates to so much more than just the physical body. It is an energetic field whereby the movement of the energy is clockwise in a healthy field and counterclockwise if the area is not balanced.

One can test the Chakras with a pendulum to see how the fields are moving in direction and strength. There are many models like this model using the energy of the body to balance the body on all levels such as acupuncture and the energy of Chi through the meridian channels. These practices are thousands of years old, much longer than the existence of western medicine.

My understanding of the chakra system helped me understand my visit with the gastroenterologist and that my stomach pain was related to the emotion of inner power. At that point in my life, I felt as though I had no power and that I had no control of my outcome.

I had studied since I was 13 years old to become a doctor and the MCAT exam was getting in the way of achieving my goals. I had pain and burning in my solar plexus area. Once my heart was open and I cried, I was then able then to get my power back.

I was accepted into medical school in late summer and would be starting in the fall, but my inner voice told me otherwise. I told my mother impromptu, without even pondering my thought, that I was not going to medical school and instead

I was going to Israel. I added that I would stay home for 6 months, re-apply and then go to Israel.

I felt like I "threw up". The words came out of my mouth without even planning this in my mind. I had no relatives, family or friends in Israel, but I knew I had to go. My mother thought I was crazy and so did the school administrators, but I was going to follow through – I was going to Israel and leaving my old world behind

So, one might ask, how could I afford to go to Israel? My parents were not supportive, especially my mother, and they were just not going to fund me. The summer of my acceptance into medical school was spent putting my artistic talent to work in Westhampton, N.Y.

I was living with six graduate girls from my college and we all intended to be waitresses. I tried waitressing at a popular Italian restaurant but hated the job. I told my dad that I was miserable, and he told me to come home. I thought about my situation and decided, why not sell all the barrettes and designed shirts I had made? But where could I sell them? The idea of selling them on the beach in the Hamptons sounded appealing.

This was at the time President Reagan was in office and people had money in the Hamptons and lots of it. The Westhampton beach had two bars, and everyone had money for drinks and food. I asked one of my roommates if she wanted to join me. She thought I was nuts and flat out said no.

The other roommate I asked was interested. Her father was a salesman and she had the sales genes in her as well. She was struggling with working as a waitress, so we were completely in agreement to make this change in our summer careers. She was also one of my mentors to get me to go to Israel as she had spent a college semester there and raved about her experiences.

We started out selling barrettes and t-shirts walking away with $75 dollars each, and then – I had another idea. Sunglasses – I thought sunglasses could really be a great seller to both men and women. We bought sunglasses wholesale to sell and by the end of the summer we each had a big fistful of cash. Enough to go to Israel and buy a car for medical school. There definitely was a higher force helping me follow my path.

CHAPTER 4

CRANIAL THERAPY

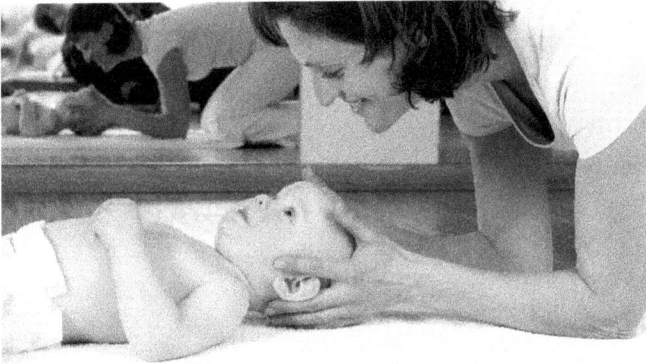

The added segment of the osteopathic curriculum that sets it apart from an allopathic medical school is its own extra course in osteopathy – the hands-on diagnoses and manipulation of the musculoskeletal system and its structural relationship to the internal organs, circulation, and lymphatic flow.

The sacrum is very much related to the neck. Here's how it works: the dura, which is a lot like the plastic wrap you store leftovers in, surrounds your brain, attaches to the upper neck and then travels down the spine, attaching to the sacrum. If the sacrum gets stuck due to trauma, it can affect the cranium (skull and what lies beneath it) and cervical spine (neck), as well as the rest of the spinal cord, through the connection of the dura.

Cranial treatment is extremely useful after trauma to the head or body, which can alter or hinder the flow of the fluids of the body. Often a trauma has dramatic, and sometimes drastic, effects on health and function.

The most obvious case is birth trauma, where the baby's skull is impacted by repeated pushing against the birth canal or by vacuum extraction or forceps delivery in difficult labor. Even an almost imperceptible alteration in skull's natural configuration and movement can lead to colic, the inability to swallow or suck, frequent spitting up, chronic ear infections, delayed development or all the above.

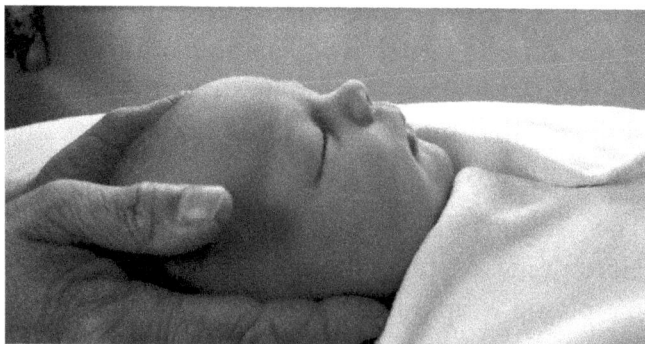

(Image: Geraldine Bright, Osteopath)

Trauma in adults can lead to low back problems, headaches, breathing problems, digestive disorders, joint pain, menstrual difficulties and repetitive stress injuries.

When I announced that I was going to Israel and deferring medical school, my mother was, of course, shocked. The plans were made. During the fall, instead of starting school, I would live at home and prepare to leave in January for an extended stay in Israel. I had to figure out where I would stay in Israel and what I would do in N.Y. while I was home for four months.

I decided I would continue selling sunglasses at various colleges either at their student unions or in the dorm rooms and at college football games. I did not make nearly as much money as I did in the Hamptons. This was just a means to make money for the moment and definitely not a career.

I made plans to volunteer in the Israeli Army through a program called Volunteers for Israel, for all age groups. I departed for Israel on New Year's Eve.

Living at home with my parents was a huge adjustment after four years of college. I kept feeling like I was falling backward into childhood. There were past issues facing me that I had blocked out as a child.

My parents always had financial issues and I was now stuck in the middle of their stressors of paying the mortgage, utilities, and food. I felt the pain of this instability and it started to affect my health. I began to have heavy, irregular menstrual cycles which occurred every 2 weeks for which I was directed to a gynecologist with a good reputation. Although I had never seen him before and a modest young 21-year-old, after taking my medical history, he asked if he could interview me for a book he was writing.

I innocently agreed, but each question was more probing and personal than the next, and I became very uncomfortable. At the time, I did not think of the word "exploitation" but I am certain as I look back, exploitation was indeed the correct term for compromising a new patient's privacy in this way.

Nor was that the end of the story. On examining me, he could find nothing wrong. However, he prescribed high doses of estrogen and sent me home. When I began to take the pills, I became violently nauseated. It was so bad, I could not function, so I called the doctor's office.

Here's what didn't happen: I was not told that the nausea was transient and would pass in three or four days. I was not told that I could take a decreased dose. Instead, the doctor's entire message was: "Do exactly as I told you." I was flabbergasted and angry. I could not take any more of the estrogen, so I tossed it and the doctor.

I then saw a second gynecologist who was kind and had me try birth control pills which did not help either. When I was three days away from going to Israel, he recommended that I have a D&C (known among doctors as a dusting and a cleaning). After this cleaning out procedure, I was off to Israel one day later.

Although I was perfectly healthy the whole time I traveled, I know now that the most important part of my "cure" was simply getting out of my childhood home and off to Israel – my longing dream come true, after four hard years of college in premedical studies.

CHAPTER 5

ISRAEL CONTINUED

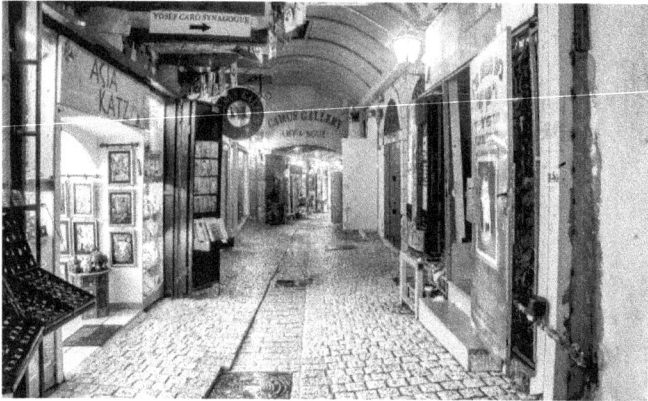

I spent five very special months in Israel and never lacked for food, clothing or shelter. For the first time in my life, I left all my self- imposed responsibilities behind and was free to travel and explore.

First, I volunteered for the Israeli Army and was sent to a tank maintenance camp where army machinery was repaired. One of the soldiers I met told me his story of seeing his closest friend in the battalion shot and killed near the Lebanese border during the Lebanese War. He had a nervous breakdown and was then sent to the maintenance camp as he could no longer endure combat emotionally.

We would have conversations about the differences between their culture and American culture. Back in the eighties, Israelis would go out to enjoy themselves without having to drink alcohol. They were appreciative of life and knew how to enjoy their free moments naturally.

From age 18 to 21, both young men and women served in the army so that by the time they were out of the army they would have a direction towards continuing education or vocational skills. It was a very practical society to me with little wasted time.

On the weekends, we could travel or spend the Sabbath nearby. Once I went with a group of volunteers to Jerusalem arriving early in the evening on a Thursday night. I was struck at once by the clear blue night sky framed by the Old City walls. It felt like I had gone back in time about 2,000 years.

Experiencing Jerusalem for the first time was beyond what I had ever imagined. On Friday evenings, we went to the Kotel (Western Wall) where people from all walks of life were praying.

The Kotel, as it is known to Israeli's faces the future building of the Third Temple. One Friday evening, three of us women volunteers were standing at the wall and we were approached there by a man who volunteered his time showing us the Old City and surroundings of Jerusalem and then placing us in homes of people that observed the Sabbath.

This was my first Sabbath (Shabbat) experience. We were placed with a Hasidic family born and raised in Jerusalem and lived in Israel for many generations. The family had eleven children.

The men sat at a different table and they all danced around the table after each course singing different traditional melodies. These melodies were (nigunim) developed by the Hasidim during times of famine in Eastern Europe to keep their spirits uplifted. It was really beautiful to see but also a very different cultural experience for me. The wife conversed with us about getting married and the importance of family.

All three of us were career oriented women not thinking consciously at the time of marriage or children. I grew up in an environment that was focused on career and financial success. My parents were closer to the value of marriage and raising children, but they chose to raise us differently especially us girls, as my mother grew up in the 1940's with limited career choices for women.

She would tell me that women in her day would graduate from high school and soon after, most would get married and have children. I remember my mother telling me that her class valedictorian was married right out of high school. I have no regrets on having a career but, I think there needs to be a balance and that no matter what – family comes first.

Women are naturally equipped to bear children and to multitask and play the directing role in the family. There are exceptions of course. I was clueless about family back then but definitely had a rude awakening once I got married years later.

Another weekend I was set up for a Sabbath on a beautiful Moshav, (Moshav is a type of agricultural community in Israel consisting of a group of individual farms. The moshav is generally based on the principle of private ownership of land, emphasis on community labor and communal marketing) south of Tel Aviv.

Each resident had their own property of fruits and vegetables that were harvested by outside workers. Most of the Moshav residents were professionals working outside of their community. They were modern orthodox meaning they lived in the times and were worldly, but they kept the traditional values of Judaism including the Sabbath.

The residents were Jews from all over the world. This place stole my heart. The family we stayed with were role models for me. The parents both had careers and a beautiful family, a home with an acre land of grapes, friendly neighbors, and community. I longed to live like this one day.

Once Volunteers for Israel was over, I went to the Jewish Agency to find out what more I could do in Israel. Choices were to work on archeological sites, learn Hebrew or learn about my Jewish heritage. I chose to go to Safed and learn about Judaism. The program was a work study program called Livnot U'lehibanot meaning "to build and to be built'. The program was going to start in three weeks, so I had time to travel beforehand.

I decided to go to Eilat, the south of Israel and the city of coral reefs, in the interim. I did have my scuba diving license and had the opportunity to finally see the most magnificent reefs in the world. I went alone and stayed in a youth hostel. I met many people from Europe and the US and even bumped into a high school friend at the youth hostel.

My sister had just lost her job and I convinced her to come to Israel. In one week, she purchased her passport and was on a plane to Israel. We chose to meet at the Western Wall in Jerusalem the following week.

While staying at the youth hostel I overheard a couple who wanted to travel to the Sinai which at that time had recently been given back to Egypt. The Sinai had one of the world's best scuba diving and snorkeling sites. I asked them if I could go with them and they agreed.

We arrived on the border of Egypt and Israel and had to get our passports checked and then we were on our way to Sharm El Sheikh in the Sinai.

On the way, we saw women walking with baskets on their heads and men on camels walking. What a different world I was seeing.

We arrived in Sharm El Sheikh and two more European travelers joined us – five in all. The place was desolate, just the exquisite turquoise, the Red Sea, the Bedouin nomads, a bar on the beach and some bathrooms. All the hotels were knocked down before the land was given back to Egypt.

There was not a soul around besides us and a few Egyptians. The skies were perfectly blue and clear, and we could see Saudi Arabia, Egypt, and Jordan from this little corner of the Middle East. Staying in this quiet, desolate place with beauty abounding, I was in heaven on earth. We all became good friends in those 5 days. We also mingled with the Egyptians who were doctors, escaping their responsibilities. They showed us their belly dancing talents and we all watched in amazement. The world under the ocean was beyond beautiful – with coral reefs of neon colors – completely magical. Sleeping under the stars in our sleeping bags was heavenly. Was I on Earth?

I knew this bliss would come to an end as I planned to meet my sister so off I went back to Jerusalem on the winding desert roads. We met at the Western Wall at exactly 5 pm. We did not have cell phones back then so exact planning was important. She traveled to Israel solo and until this day she is not sure how she made it to Jerusalem on her own. She ended up at a youth hostel in Tel Aviv with some Scandinavians she met at the airport. She then boarded a train guided by an Israeli who said it would be the most scenic route to Jerusalem.

There was only one train that left for Jerusalem from Tel Aviv, so she waited half a day for that train. There was only one other passenger on the train – an Israeli soldier. He guided her in Hebrew and took her to the Western Wall himself.

When we met, she hardly recognized me as I was so tanned. We hugged each other, reunited in our land. She too felt like she was home and we were both misty-eyed. We were approached by a Jewish religious woman who asked us if we needed a place to stay as we looked like the proverbial backpackers. She showed us to the Old City of Jerusalem in the Jewish Quarter and invited us into a beautiful youth hostel.

Before you know it, we were escorted by an older man to a school to learn about the existence of G-d and the principles of Judaism. We enjoyed the classes and we met wonderful young women mostly from abroad. Our discussions were G-d focused and what better place to be than in Jerusalem to be talking about G-d and our relationship with the creator.

We soon joined the program in Safed learning about and working on the restoration of archeological sites and helping the Ethiopians immigrate into Israel after Operation Moses.

Safed is a magical place with old stone attached homes and blue arched doors facing the holy site of Mount Meron. Many important Jewish sages are buried there, but Meron is most well-known as the burial site of Rabbi Shimon bar Yochai.

Rabbi Shimon, who lived in the 2nd century CE, was the first to publicly teach the mystical dimension of the Torah known as the Kabbalah and is the author of the basic work of Kabbalah, the Zohar. Every year, on the anniversary of Rabbi Shimon's passing, hundreds of thousands converge in Meron for a joyous celebration of his life and the revelation of the esoteric soul of Torah.

The air was crisp, and the city dotted with ancient, gnarled olive trees. I was impressed by the simplistic nature of the place. If I asked for directions the answer would be to make a left by the orange tree and a right at the lemon tree and then go straight toward the olive tree and you will see it on the right.

Little did we know, we were in the Kabbalistic center of Israel. Safed was the home of the great holy sages, many who were Kabbalists from earlier centuries that lie below the city in graves intermingled with caves that were used for meditation. Safed was very expansive to the mind. There was an artist colony which made perfect sense as the atmosphere there was conducive to creativity and expansiveness.

The holy gravesites intrigued me. One day I decided to take a walk down to the cemetery and past the graves. The land was expansive and beautiful with white rocks jutting out of the ground and wildflowers of varied colors interspersed. It was quiet and peaceful.

I could think so clearly and vividly imagine Abraham or our first forefather with sheep grazing in these pastures. I was pleasantly lost somewhere back in time. Many times I went beyond the grave sites and took a paper and pen and would draw, feeling so free to be creative.

Back at our program, we were building a synagogue from the ruins. We learned how to mix cement, throw it on the walls and then smooth it out with a scraper. We mostly made a mess and the builder in charge fixed all our mistakes.

We learned how to keep kosher which was not too hard as we each took turns cooking only vegetarian food. This way we would not have issues with mixing milk with meat. We would escape at times and get falafel or shawarma in town.

In the afternoon we learned about various Jewish topics including history, the Torah portion of the week, the prophets, kings, Jewish holidays and

Jewish law. We had very open and caring instructors and I found the learning very meaningful. I decided after leaving this program that I would slowly continue learning and growing in Judaism and spirituality.

We had wonderful experiences on this program including a three-day walk from the Kinneret (Sea of Galilee) to the Mediterranean, from east to west, resting for lunch and finding natural pools of water to swim in. We walked through time seeing history unfolding before us as we viewed the different archeological sites we encountered.

We finally walked through a banana field and towards the Mediterranean Sea in the north of Israel. This trek was difficult at times and not all of us were able to complete the hike. My sister and I ran towards the sea and jumped in with glee.

We spent time with the Ethiopians teaching them about the holidays that were not included in the written Torah (Old Testament) such as Purim and Chanukah. In exchange, they taught us African dancing. They shared their stories of walking through the Sudan and escaping death. They were miraculously airlifted to Israel, 1000 people on a plane at a time, like stuffed sardines.

My sister and I finished the rest of our stay in Jerusalem at the original school we were learning at when my sister arrived. I knew that I would be going back to NY and sitting for years learning medicine, so I took one more trip with a friend to Egypt and the Sinai before going back.

It was very hot at the time in Egypt and the city of Cairo was swarming with people. We took a one-hour camel ride into the desert to see pyramids and on our way, we saw how the third world lived. The children and adults were carrying water from wells and they lived in huts.

How spoiled is our American culture? We could never imagine living without air conditioning and water, gas and electric. The camel ride was uncomfortable, and I would never have the desire to ride one again. I must admit – I would rather drive a car.

I left Israel with the thought that one day I would want to live in my homeland. I cried like a baby when I said goodbye to Israel as I boarded the plane. My sister was definitely there for me to help get me on that plane, otherwise, I am not sure I would have gone back to the USA. My heart was broken. I had completely fallen in love with the land and the people.

CHAPTER 6

OSTEOPATHIC MEDICAL SCHOOL

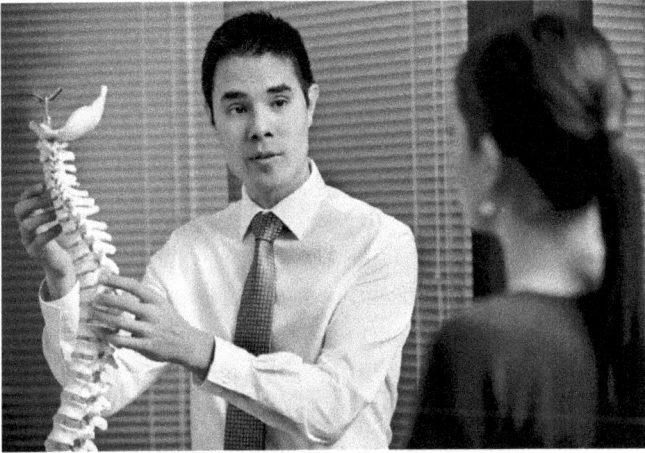

Nancy, a 45-year-old woman came into my office complaining of pain in her neck that radiated down her left arm. During the history taking I always ask if there is any history of trauma. It turned out she had fallen off her porch onto her buttocks five years before coming to see me. After the fall she had low back pain for a few days and then it subsided.

While I treated her, it felt as if her sacrum (the lowest segment of the low back below the lumbar spine) was stuck in a forward position. It simply did not move when I palpated for the motion of the sacrum. Humans are about 80% fluid and a trained Osteopath can feel the movement of this fluid in different parts of the body. It feels like a wave turning and twisting about. The amplitude of motion varies in people from strong to weak as one palpates. This movement comes from the production of Cerebrospinal Fluid in the brain that is produced and reabsorbed and has its own rate of movement per minute which is a separate rate from our arterial pulse or our respiratory rate. This rate is called the primary respiratory mechanism.

I started slowly easing the sacrum forward into the position it wanted to be in and after several minutes of treatment the sacrum suddenly released and started to move. The patient spontaneously jumped into alertness and said,

---

"what was that"? I was surprised at her spontaneous release as well and told her that her sacrum finally started to move, and she felt that shift.

She returned for a follow-up a week later. The pain in her neck was completely gone.

Very few people know much about osteopathy, yet osteopathic medical schools are springing up all over the country. In fact, the philosophy of treating the "whole person" approach has made osteopathy the fastest-growing segment of healthcare in the United States and osteopaths have become health care providers for over 20% of the population of physicians.

Harlem is a fitting location for the Touro College of Osteopathic Medicine. Many osteopathic schools have an added mission: to dispatch doctors to poorer neighborhoods and towns most in need of medical care.

I was an osteopathic preceptor in the first class in Harlem in 2007 and I am the only one left from that first class still teaching in the hospitals to the 3rd year students. They chose me because I was board certified in neuromuscular medicine and family medicine. I had never taught osteopathic students before, but I had lectured previously to the public and educated them on osteopathy. I guess gymnasts are not quitters. I hung in there through many changes in the department in the first few years in a new school. I am so glad I pursued teaching at TouroCOM as I realized how rewarding it was and how much I learned from my students, too.

Inside, Touro seems indistinguishable from a conventional medical school – what doctors of osteopathic Medicine, or D.O.s, call allopathic, a term that some M.D.s aren't fond of.

A walk through the corridors finds students practicing skills on mannequins, hard-wired with faulty hearts. They dissect cadavers. They bend over lab tables, working with professors on their research.

And, unlike their allopathic counterparts, they spend roughly five hours a week being instructed in the century-old techniques of osteopathic medicine which include manipulating the spine, muscles, fascia, fluid and bones in diagnosis and treatment. In one classroom, several students lay flat on examining tables while classmates learn hands- on "Manipulative Therapy."

It should be noted that getting into osteopathic school is still excruciatingly tough. Imagine

16,500 students applying for some 6,400 spots. Touro has received 6,000 applications for 270 first-year seats for the Manhattan school and their campus in Middletown, N.Y.

The boom in osteopathy is striking. In 1980, there were just 14 schools across the country and 4,940 students. There are now 30 schools, including state universities in New Jersey, Ohio, Oklahoma, Texas, West Virginia and Michigan, offering instruction at 40 different locations to more than 23,000 students. Today, osteopathic schools turn out about 22 percent of the nation's medical school graduates.

Whatever the reasons for choosing a D.O. over an M.D. degree, osteopathic medicine has, for decades now and increasingly so, been accepted as authoritative training by the medical establishment, including the residency programs that lead to licensure.

About 60 percent of D.O. graduates go on to primary care fields like internal medicine, pediatrics and family medicine, compared with about 30 percent of M.D.s.

Osteopathic skills were first consolidated by a 19th-century frontier physician, who returned from serving as a physician in the Civil War, had become dissatisfied with the state of the medical profession.

Andrew Taylor Still, who decried the overuse of

arsenic, castor oil, opium, and elixirs and believed that many diseases had their roots in a disturbed musculoskeletal system that could be treated hands on. He founded the first osteopathic school in 1892 in Kirksville, Mo. – A.T. Still University.

In the late 19th Century, there were basically three schools of thought around healing - homeopathy, allopathy, and eclectic medicine.

Homeopathy, established by Samuel Hahnemann is based on prescribing microscopic doses of medicines that produce the same symptoms as the disease to assist the body's own healing response.

Allopathy is the most common form of medicine practiced today. Its practitioners are MDs whose therapy relies on drugs and surgery to cure diseases.

The eclectic school borrowed from many healing traditions and was likely to vary from practitioner to practitioner.

Dr. Still disliked using drugs. He had observed that whenever he found disease in a patient he also found problems in the musculoskeletal system. He thought imbalances in the circulatory, lymphatic and nervous systems caused the problems, and solved it by manipulating the body with his hands to treat restrictions in the body and therefore restore health. He coined the term osteo- (Greek for bone) pathy (Greek for suffering).

At the heart of osteopathy is a holistic approach: health and well-being are believed to depend on the maintenance of all the body's related systems. The osteopath helps to realign the body so that it can heal itself.

Unlike most allopaths, an osteopath is as concerned about why there is a problem in the musculoskeletal system as with the physical symptoms the patient is presenting. The osteopath delves into the patient's lifestyle and mental and emotional health as part of the treatment. The added segment of osteopathic curriculum that sets it apart from an allopathic medical school is instruction in the hands-on manipulation of the musculoskeletal system.

Critics have, from time to time, assailed the osteopathic techniques as a pseudoscience, though the medical establishment has come to accept the approach. And osteopathic schools offer the same academic subjects as traditional medical schools and the same two years of clinical rotations. Osteopathic schools turn out 22 percent of the nation's medical school graduates; 73,000 are now practicing physicians, more than double the number in 1990.

But an image problem remains. A recent survey by the American Osteopathic Association found that 29 percent of adults were unaware that D.O.s are licensed to practice medicine, 33 percent didn't know they can prescribe medicine and 63 percent didn't know they can perform surgery.

CHAPTER 7

DR. SARNO

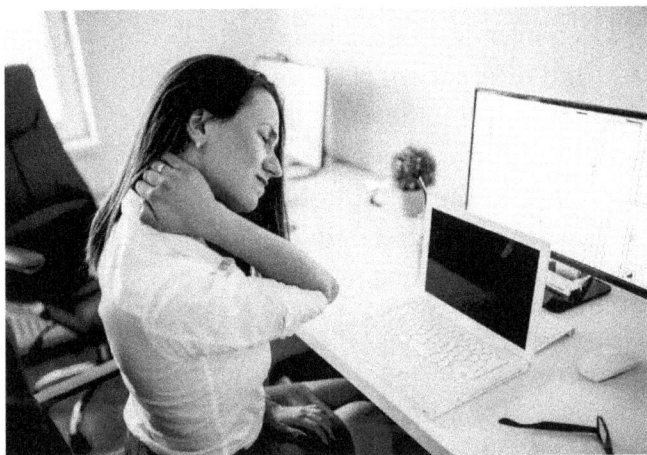

I have seen from personal experience that many doctors – especially those limited by a view of the human body as a set of separate organs and who rely exclusively on lab tests and drug therapies – are simply unequipped to treat all patients. They dismiss those whose needs overwhelm them and abandon those who cannot benefit from the limited menu of therapies most allopathic practitioners have to offer.

There is no "bedside manner" training at medical school. There are no tests that determine the E.Q. (emotional intelligence) of a physician, unfortunately. We are screened only for intellectual intelligence and therefore, common sense and "street smarts" are not considered by many doctors in making their decision.

In life, sometimes it is the small easy questions and answers that are glossed over. Anything glossed over can have a huge impact on the health and life of a patient. Doctors usually don't compare labs from the time the patient enters the hospital till the present moment and even if the lab value is slightly lower than it should be for that particular person it could be very low for their normal. You don't need to be a genius to compare labs, but you do need to be dedicated.

For example, when my mother went into the hospital with a history of leukemia and suffering from a stomach virus, her labs that determine how anemic she was when she came into the hospital were a little low.

When I asked the hospitalist the next day how her labs were, he said they were a little low. I then asked the specific count and she had dropped 2 points in one day which is highly important in determining whether she needed a blood transfusion. I had to reprimand the on-call physician, saying that my mother could die, between the drop in blood count and the stomach virus, if she was not transfused.

We are also not told how to speak to a patient when all lab values and studies are normal, but the patient does not feel well. In western medicine, we learn that a patient can be malingering, meaning that they are lying about their illness. Most people do not lie about how they feel.

Health professionals need to learn how to say they understand and to be empathetic – and assure their patients that there are modalities of treatments that may help them. First, the doctor has to be open-minded and humble to learn about the alternatives to western medicine and then the doctor can either learn some of these alternative treatments or refer patients to another practitioner well versed in their modality of treatment.

Examples of other practices and philosophies of healing other than western medicine just to name a few are – osteopathy, chiropractic, homeopathy, herbs, nutritional health, ayurvedic medicine, and acupuncture. Within these specific areas, there are also different philosophies of practice and different treatment modalities. For example, there are different styles and schools of acupuncture such as Traditional Chinese Medicine (TCM), Japanese Meridian, Korean hand, and Five Element acupuncture to name a few.

Within these different schools of acupuncture, the tools that are used may vary such as needle sizing, various types of moxibustion, manaka hammer, ear acupuncture, magnets at meridian points, cupping, Gua Sha (scraping technique) and laser.

Acupuncture is an ancient form of medicine looking deeper into the individual at the level of body, mind, and spirit. Whereas western medicine focuses on the physical component only and is newly developed in comparison.

Wouldn't it be nice if we could use the best of both worlds and be humble enough to know that not everyone heals the same way?

A doctor needs to be supportive of the patient on all levels: physical, emotional, and spiritual. In medical school, I was "indoctrinated" on how to use science, but not how to use my own intuition. As I saw more and more patients, however, I began to realize that rote knowledge was not going to solve all their problems.

Over time, I developed a sense of the balance of art and science, data and intuition. I began to be able to "read between the lines," As I spoke with my patients. I would ask questions delving into their past such as their childhood, their current stressors, the foods they craved or avoided, and the exercises they did and how often.

I found it was important to ask about physical, mental and emotional traumas, including birth trauma. Even dental work can yield important clues about a patient's tendencies toward infections and inflammation.

For example, braces may be traumatic for a patient if it is changing the structure of their palate as the palate is connected to higher structures that are connected to the pituitary gland – the "master gland" that controls all the hormones in the body. These hormones can thus affect the nervous system and the immune system as all these systems are all interconnected.

It is also important to learn more than a patient's job title. I ask about their work environment, how much they work and their mode of working – is he/ she a perfectionist, a people pleaser? Is he/she a workaholic? Does she/he have a hateful boss?

Many times, I refer my patients to read John Sarno's, M.D. books if they are pressured internally or externally. If they have physical pain they may be diverting their emotional subconscious rage to physical pain and not aware or acknowledging their anger. Such creative and sneaky systems we have!

The treatment that Dr. Sarno explains is to acknowledge the anger and sometimes they must take it a step further and seek psychoanalytical therapist if their childhood foundation was unstable. The process of acknowledging anger takes consistency and time and is highly recommended for those with pain who are not getting better by other modalities of treatment or if they fit the "Sarno Picture." Of course, physical pathology is ruled out first.

CASE STUDIES

Norman was a 68-year-old male who called me right before a big holiday and told me that he was lying on the floor in excruciating pain. He did not know how he was going to get up and he wanted me to give him an injection to alleviate his pain.

I happened to be reading Dr. Sarno's book, "The Body-Mind Connection – Healing the Body Healing the Pain", for the 2nd time when I received Norman's phone call. I went to his home, a syringe with an anesthetic in hand, just in case. There he was lying on the floor unable to get up.

I did some neurological testing which was normal, and I palpated his low back and took his history. He told me that he was bending down to pick something up and his back had gone out. The pain came on suddenly. He did have muscle tightness in his low back. I told him that as soon as he was able to move, we would order an X-ray and possibly an MRI of his low back.

I then started asking him about stressors in his life. He responded with an emphatic "yes" to many stressors. His father-in-law just had passed on as well as his best friend and he had a pressured business that was in financial upheaval. I asked him how he felt about getting older. He was scared, especially after his close friend passed on. He was frustrated about his business as well. I asked him if he was a "people pleaser" and he said yes. He also said he was a perfectionist and hard on himself.

I then gave him an injection for pain relief and told him to start reading Dr. Sarno's book. He was stuck on his back anyway, so he said, "why not". He read and read and talked to himself daily on the specific frustrations that he had and in two weeks he was completely better.

He took the book very seriously as if it were the bible and really worked on bringing his unconscious rage

*into consciousness and acknowl-
edged specific events and matters in
life that made him angry. Whenever
Norman would get a twinge of pain
he would think of what was making
him upset or angry and the pain
would go away. He called me his
Sarno Rebbe. He never went to a
chiropractor again. He was a classic
Sarno type.*

*Dean was another Sarno story. A
65-year-old man diagnosed with kidney cancer and in need of surgery.
He came to my office very noncha-
lant about his condition. He told me
that his back was hurting and that he
had diarrhea and an irritable bowel.
I sensed that he was blocking out his
current cancer diagnosis and his repressed anger was being expressed
by physical pain. I told Dean to read
Dr. Sarno's book, "Healing Back
Pain: The Mind-Body Connection".*

*Dean followed his instruction to talk
to himself about what was making
him angry and tell himself that his
mind was creating the pain as a
diversion from the fear of cancer.
He yelled at it to stop. And that it*

was unnecessary.

He yelled and yelled, "Stop it. Stop the pain. You don't need to do this."

In about thirty minutes, he got up and was able to walk and the pain was gone. It returned a day or two later. He went through the process again and the pain disappeared again. There was a third episode that he controlled the same way. The pain never recurred.

Larry was a 40-year-old man who was single who was suffering from low back pain with radiating pain down his left leg and walked with a foot drop (he was unable to lift his foot up properly when walking so it dragged). He was diagnosed with 3 disc herniations of the low back and then was told that nerve blocks and physical therapy would help him, so he took that course of action only to be still in pain months later.

I had known Larry for many years as a friend and I asked him the classic "Sarno" questions. Are you a "people pleaser"? Do you put a lot of pressure on yourself? Do you like to look good in other people's eyes? He said yes to all and then I proceeded to tell him about Dr. Sarno's books and I lent him the book.

He was so impressed that he went to Dr. Sarno in NYC. and after walking out of his lecture his pain went away. "Are you serious"? I asked, "you had relief that fast?" He joined the support groups and became totally free from his pain. Whenever he would have a twinge of pain he would whip out his cd's and listen and then the pain would stop. He was cured.

How did I even get to learn about Dr. Sarno? One of my patients had told me that her back pain completely went away when reading and going to see Dr. Sarno. She was in bed with back pain for months and Dr. Sarno's method worked for her.

I read his books and became a fan. I decided to call Dr. Sarno and asked him if I could spend a few days watching him treat patients in his office. He was agreeable and told me that he wished more doctors were open minded like me and learn his method of healing.

I had spent three days with him watching him make his diagnosis of tension myositis by taking a good history, including stressors of life and exploring their personality type and palpating various points on the body that relate to tension myositis. Dr. Sarno palpated the back of the head, the neck, top of the shoulders (trapezius muscle), low back, buttock (piriformis and gluteal muscles), and the outside of the legs (the iliotibial band). All his patients had most of these tender points. The patients then went to watch him lecture.

For some of the patients who had serious childhood issues, he recommended psychoanalytical therapy. He also offered a support group that I attended. All of Dr. Sarno's patients suffered from chronic pain. All had had previous X-rays and MRI's before being selected as a "Sarno" candidate.

For me, Dr. Sarno's books touched a strong emotional core that I needed to act upon. So, I contacted him, and he arranged for me to see patients with him. At the time, I was personally in the lowest state of my life. Everything around me was falling apart and so was I.

I had just had my 5th child and before that, I had been an insomniac for three years due to being totally torn between working and being the mother of four children. I yearned to be home with my children which brought up my own childhood issue of being emotionally neglected while my mom worked full time. My mother was absent for comfort during my times of illness or personal crises. My mother's story growing up with an abusive, overbearing and controlling father, did not allow her to be a child. My grandfather restricted her freedom to play with her friends outside the home.

It was difficult for my mother to meet the emotional responsibility of being a parent. She had a need to go out, enjoy herself with friends and be the carefree child that she missed out on. I remember my therapist telling me that neglect can be emotionally damaging, even more so than abuse.

I wanted to be there for my children and nurture them, but I was in conflict. Financially, I had no choice but to work. I did not know how to delegate responsibility to my five boys or my husband, because I was raised independently and did everything for myself.

I continued this path of pushing myself to be the perfect mom doing most everything on my own – from shopping to cooking to cleaning to caretaking. I did have a live-in cleaning lady to care for my youngest boy while I was working. I must admit, it was so painful to leave my youngest son home with her when I went to work.

I wore myself into the ground physically getting sick frequently during my pregnancy and postpartum with my fourth child. While I was six months pregnant, I vividly remember that I had to take a course for the neuromuscular medicine board to be proficient in osteopathic techniques. The plane was leaving at 8 am. The morning before I began having symptoms of urinary frequency and pain on urination. I started taking an antibiotic, but it was not working so I called a nearby pharmacist and he was nice enough to deliver the medication himself on his way home from work.

I did not know at that time how to rest and listen to my body. I just kept pushing myself to my limit. I did get better and the course went well but I could never do that now looking back.

I took the Osteopathic Neuromuscular Medicine proficiency board exams six months after my fourth son was born. My son, our caretaker, and I flew to Indianapolis to take the boards and on the way from the airport to the hotel, a truck hit the limousine we were traveling in.

We were all fine physically, but my nervous system was in shock. I had to pull myself together to take a three-hour exam immediately after arriving at the hotel. When I came back home I was not quite the same. This is when insomnia began and lasted for three years.

The icing on the cake was after my fifth child was

born. We had two major crises at work. I was working in both a no-fault / worker's compensation practice one day a week and I had my own integrative practice four days a week.

I was a naive idealist. The practice included a hypnotherapist, another osteopath, an acupuncturist, a classical homeopath, a physical therapist, a nutritionist, a massage therapist and a Rolfer. I would initially see the patient and then I would treat and refer to other practitioners according to their condition and what I believed would help them best. I was successful with helping patients, but the rent was very high and most of our earnings went back into the practice.

One day the hypnotherapist decided to start his own practice in the same building on the same floor as my practice and take my existing patients with him. We did not have a non- compete clause due to ignorance on my part. The hypnotherapist and the other osteopath decided that they would work together. I felt betrayed and angry. I felt I had no choice but to find a new place to work. I did not want to be a victim.

The owners of the building were lawyers and tough ones at that. They told me that I would have to pay over $30,000 to break my lease. I did not have this kind of money, so I had to declare bankruptcy which was humiliating.

We moved to another location and I started to

have severe pain in my forearms. I could not sleep, had palpitations, nausea, sensitivity to light and sound and basically, I was done, but the trauma continued.

A man walked into my office one day and gave me a subpoena that was related to the no fault practice for medical misconduct. What did I do wrong, I asked? They said it was about the man I was working for.

I then found out that the manager was committing insurance fraud using my name from a signed stamper he had stolen. I had no idea he was billing insurance companies double and triple the amount. I was practicing for 10 years and I was so ignorant and uneducated in this area.

This was not something on the radar in medical school back in the 80's. I was punished for medical misconduct for not overseeing this evil man. I then spent six months in court testifying against him and spending time at the N.Y. Department of Health being tortured by having to look at all the charts that I wrote.

I had left the no fault practice months prior to the subpoena after my fifth child was born because I had had enough and was not getting paid. This man kept telling me that the insurance companies were not paying but that I would soon get paid – which never happened.

My husband kept asking me to hang on and being

such a "people pleaser" – I did. After my baby was born, I quit, wanting to move forward from this toxic, frustrating practice. Moving forward after the subpoena, he went to jail, and I was told I could never take insurance from workers compensation or no-fault patients.

The big stressor here was that this no-fault manager approached my husband and me in my private practice to see if I would work in his practice only one-half day a week. We were so gullible, thinking this part time work would help me pay off my student loans.

Why did this man walk into my life? Really to change it forever. I eventually hit the wall and crashed. This was for me the beginning of consciousness and wisdom. Sometimes to go up in life you have to hit rock bottom. I was still sliding on the slippery slope down.

While my life was in process of being turned upside down, I proceeded to study for my family practice boards. I tuned out the chaos of which I was not in control of and studied. We tend to repeat our past.

As a child, I grew up in a very chaotic financial environment. My father was a salesman and my mom worked two jobs. They barely had enough money to pay the mortgage and the utilities, and many times water or electric was turned off without warning.

I was always living under this duress and my survival mechanism was to tune out the chaos and study and do gymnastics. I did a good job tuning out and only when the trauma recurred as an adult, could I no longer block it out anymore.

I studied all my life to be a doctor and to get out of my financial woes only to be slapped in the face with bankruptcy, my practice falling apart and the health department deciding what they were going to do with me and my license.

I brought my sister along to watch my baby while I took my boards. When the boards were over, I went into a tunnel of "death". I felt like I was dying. I asked my sister, an acupuncturist, to help. She did her magic and got me out of that acute state and I was able to go back home in one piece but very weak. I somehow passed the boards.

When I returned home, I felt vulnerable, shaky and could not sleep. I had acupuncture treatments, cranial treatments, hypnotherapy, therapy, supplements, nutrition – and I was still not sleeping. I was on my way to having a nervous breakdown. Yes, I was hitting rock bottom.

I had been to three psychiatrists and the medications gave me side effects. I felt like a guinea pig trying this and that, but I knew in my gut that I needed something specific even though no one around me thought so.

I finally got a lead from three different people to

see this one psychopharmacologist in NYC and I went. He really listened to my story and my history and gave me medication to raise my serotonin levels and to help me sleep. I was really an acute emergency room case. I was willing to try this medication because I desperately wanted to get my life back and care for my children.

After the first dose, I slept for the first time in years. The medication turned me around about 75% and in time I decreased it to half of the original dose and continued to exercise regularly, take supplements, and lead a balanced life.

I had gone for cognitive and psychoanalytic therapy for a few years to learn to understand my patterns and to feel my pain and grow from it. The most important message I got from my therapist was that if I am in a car and I move over then everyone else has to move over. Meaning, if I change, then everyone else around me will change... and thus began the work of change.

After spending time with Dr. Sarno, I decided that I was going to stop working and give myself time to do repressed anger work.

It was hard for me to "let go" because I did not know how we were going to survive financially and I was so fearful of putting my children through the chaos I went through as a child. I relied on a higher force at this point and I let go.

Once I stopped working, the emotional work

began, and it was probably the hardest and most painful process of my life... much more than any physical pain – even giving birth. I had to go back in time and feel the abandonment and chaos I had blocked out for so long.

It was a long journey leading up to my nervous breakdown. I had mononucleosis in college, was pre-med while on the gymnastics team in college, went to medical school and was pregnant during my fourth year of medical school and the first year of internship fifteen months apart, had four children and was the sole provider, and had many infections during my pregnancy. After my fourth child was born I experienced multiple episodes of strep throat, urinary tract infections, and viral meningitis.

I just kept going as this was my pattern. A pattern most likely formed from gymnastics, a sport that had me pushing myself to my limits with ripped skin on my hands, shin splints, bruised hips, sprains, and many falls.

My journey to health was a process that included many modalities of treatment and my own inner work. My chest pain and palpitations stopped when I started natural hormone replacement therapy because both my estrogen and progesterone were low at the age of thirty-eight. Taking these hormones allowed me to lower the doses of the medication in half.

Acupuncture and herbs helped my immune system get stronger. Homeopathy stopped my chronic fatigue states when I would have swollen glands, malaise and a need to rest for days.

The homeopath gave me a remedy that fits a "stock broker type," that runs and runs and then crashes. Acupuncture addressed my fire and wood element, with treatments along the meridians for the liver/gallbladder and circulation.

My nature is fiery – always on the run as well as a planner/organizer type and repressed anger – the wood element (gallbladder and liver) in the acupuncture model. It took me many years to learn how to pace myself and not overdo it. Sounds so easy, but it is so hard at least for me, "the fiery one".

Over the years, cranial therapy, Rolfing and massage helped my nervous system relax and healed physical pain. I had many physical traumas as a child and adult. I had braces and a night guard for four years. I was injured many times as a gymnast, experiencing a severe concussion, severe ankle sprain needing crutches, and a couple of whiplash injuries.

During my healing process, I chose to learn about yoga and became certified as a yoga instructor. I also took a workshop to become a certified JourneyDance™ instructor and an Ayurvedic course at Kripalu in Massachusetts. This all helped me with understanding myself, taught me to eat right for my body type, gave me joy and taught me to meditate and breathe correctly as a daily practice.

There is always a positive that comes from difficult experiences if you chose to look deep enough. When my nervous system was really weak I noticed that if I walked a block I would feel my cranial mechanism moving in my brain and my head would pound. I would then rest and feel the fluid moving in my brain and observed my whole nervous system unwind and slow down as I rested.

Resting was very helpful to my recovery and the more I gave myself space to just be in the moment, the better I started to feel.

I began practicing being in the moment when going food shopping. I focused on the item that I put in my cart and then the next item and so on. Totally staying in the moment was so beneficial at that point enabling me to slow down and feel stronger. I could not think ahead at that point.

There was something good to say about really being in the present and experiencing it. I worked on not projecting into the future or I would go into a fearful place. Even when I was weak and unable to walk without feeling physical pain, I stayed in the moment as much as I could.

I learned from cranial courses from Dr. Sutherland's quotes. "Be still and know that I am your

G-d." (Tehillim or psalms 46:10) written by King David. I learned slowly to be in stillness in an osteopathic way, a spiritual way, and an emotional way. I was still... and I knew that G-d was above me.

We don't want or ask to be sick or in hardship, but when it happens it can be a great opportunity to cling to a source far greater than us for help, healing, guidance and protection.

CHAPTER 8

MY INTERNSHIP AND BEYOND

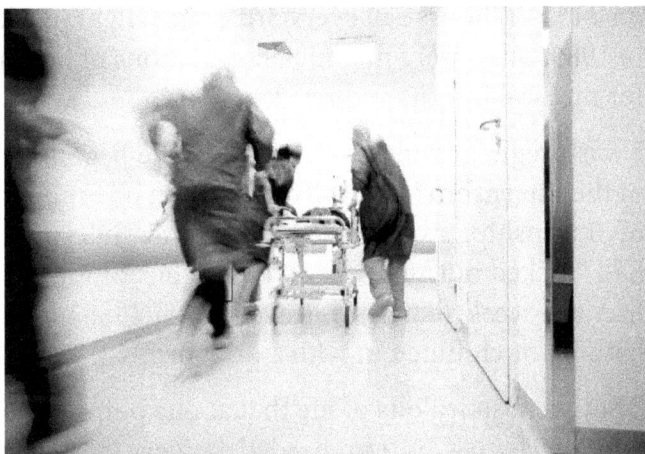

My first year as an intern was an experience of a lifetime. I was working in Rockaway, NY, in a hospital in an inner-city area with many nursing homes, in a MASH unit – literally.

We saw gunshot and stab wounds, very sick AIDS patients, elderly patients in a fetal position and everything in between. I felt so pained at times that I had to learn to block the pain and protect my heart creating a numb like feeling.

There were no resident physicians above us except in surgery so if there was a problem we had to call the attending physician. Of course, they did not like us to call them, especially at 3 am. We were running the show along with the nurses. Notes did not count that much but saving lives did.

All the residents were in survival mode as we were on 24 to 36 hours call every 3rd or 4th night. Back in 1989, there were no official regulations of hours for medical interns and residents.

I was pregnant with my first son in the beginning of the internship and gave birth within one month of internship. According to the other interns, I had "lucked out" and they were jealous of me as I had a 6-week maternity leave – as if I was sun-bathing or chilling out with a newborn.

They were so jealous of me that at one point when another female intern needed surgery and was going to end her internship 6 weeks early, they wanted me to fill in for her on-call nights.

I told them that they were living in the 1920's as women now had maternity rights and it was in my contract. I was about to call a lawyer if they continued their assertion of me filling her spot at night. I had enough on-calls of my own to deal with.

This was a "survival of the fittest" internship. The first day returning to work I saw my maternal instincts in action. I cried as I did not want to leave my baby and return to ICU with long and hard hours. I was pregnant again 6 months later and working over 80 hours a week.

It was not in my plans to have another child so quickly but so much for plans. My second born was a stoic survivor of half of the internship and the second year of residency. He was born 9 days late even though statistically interns give birth 6 weeks early due to the stressors of the internship. To this day – he is strong, determined, and resilient.

My war stories of internship and residency that stand out till this day are:

My encounter with life and death of two people at the same time on a Sunday while doing a 12-hour shift. One man with emphysema washaving seizures and I was instructed to give him three rounds of injections of anti-seizure medication every 15 minutes, while another patient had an intestinal obstruction and I needed to insert a nasogastric (NG) tube down her nose.

I could not get this tube down her nose after many tries and I had to keep thinking of injecting the other patient on time. I called the house officer and he came down to insert the nasogastric tube. He shoved it down her nose and then pumped air into her belly with a syringe attached to the tubing.

He said he heard air sounds in her belly when he pumped the air in. I listened as well but I did not hear air sounds. He was confident with the insertion and walked away. I wasn't feeling as confident, so I kept checking up on her and before you know it she stopped breathing.

Thank G-d a pulmonary doctor happened to be in the hospital as her lung collapsed because the nasogastric tube had gone into her lung instead of her stomach. The pulmonologist inserted a chest tube into her lung, so she survived the ordeal. The house officer and I had to write notes explaining the situation as this was caused by the house officer's poor judgment.

In the meantime, the seizing patient was transferred to ICU and I had to write transfer notes as well. The nurses on the floor above me were calling me saying that 30 IV's and labs had to be done. I remember being overwhelmed and telling the nurses to call another resident because I needed help. Of course, the other resident was angry that he had to do extra work.

Another time, I remember an obese intern being ordered by the attending doctor to draw blood gasses on a patient every 30 minutes which was a bit excessive as the patient was on a ventilator. The intern was sweating profusely from running back and forth getting these blood gasses. The intern totally "lost it" from overwork.

He put the ventilator on maximum capacity and stormed out and said, "now I don't have to draw any more blood gasses." Drawing a blood gas means you have to use a needle to draw blood from an artery in the wrist. The resident was maxed out and so was the patient.

The next story involves myself and an emergency room nurse getting stuck in the elevator with an emergency room patient who had pneumonia. This patient was supposed to be transferred to the ICU. We were stuck in the elevator for an hour and I was 7 months pregnant.

The patient needed oxygen which was forgotten on the gurney, so the gas tank was raised up through the shaft of the elevator until it reached us. I remember so clearly that it was 2 a.m. and that maybe they would have pity on me and let me rest for a while when they got the door open. Unfortunately, no.

After an hour, the fire department came and pried the elevator door open and had us climb down on a ladder to the floor below and then hoisted the patient on the gurney down as well.

I was free for one second and then I got a call on my beeper from the resident covering me in the ICU." Where are you? Get down here right now. I was covering your patients while you were in the elevator." I replied, "I just went to get a drink of water." My unborn child went through the mill as I was so stressed out.

My most crucial personal story was making a moral and ethical decision that was a calling way higher than myself to stop the internship. I was on call in the ICU as a second-year resident. At this point, I was on call every other night for two weeks because I had to make up calls that were covered for me while I observed the Jewish Holidays.

I was completely exhausted, and sleep deprived. The nurse called me into the ICU to evaluate a patient who had a myocardial infarction (heart attack) for pain. I told the nurse to give him morphine and she did. She called again thirty minutes later and said that the patient was still in pain, so I told her to repeat the morphine.

She then said, "don't you think you should come into the ICU and check on the patient". I agreed with her. At that moment I realized staying with the internship was not fair to a patient who has a sleep-deprived intern making decisions nor to my child for whom I was absent and not giving him the care he needed. I was torn at every level: I could not be a "good doctor or a good mom".

I made the decision to take a leave of absence and wait one more month to have my second baby. If a doctor cannot have empathy toward a patient, then he or she is in the wrong field.

I decided that I would not continue with the residency in family medicine based on my ethical decision. I said to myself, "when I die I don't want to be accountable for not treating this patient properly and possibly harming him and not being involved in raising my children." I knew I would not be able to live with myself if I continued on this path.

I was very blessed that I was not obligated to finish a residency to get board certification in family medicine. My other alternative was to work for 5 years and then study for the Boards in family medicine and that is the route I chose. The year after I had finished the residency the rules changed, and one was required to finish a residency in family medicine to practice. I lucked out, but there are no coincidences. The decision I made was the right one.

My way was best for me. I practiced in walk-in clinics, hospitals, at a college and a primary care practice for two years. I had enough time to read and learn and I was not sleep deprived. The decision was hard but then it was smooth sailing from there. I took courses in osteopathy and went to integrative medicine conventions.

I always brought my children with me and a caretaker to help. I was motivated to learn as much about osteopathy and nutrition as possible and to become a successful physician ready to heal patients with as many tools as possible.

My most positive and memorable experience during my internship year began with reading a book about "Operation Moses," the exodus of the

Ethiopian Jews to Sudan and secret emergency airlifts to the USA and Israel.

These Ethiopian Jews had learned the written Torah (Old Testament) and practiced its written law for over a thousand years. The Ethiopian ruler wanted to kill the Jews. They left en masse through the rainforests to Sudan and were then hidden by Sudanese residents until the airlifts arrived. Many were separated from their families and did not survive.

I was on call and I just had finished the book that night. The next morning, I was given new patients during my surgery rotation. I walked into the room of my first new patient to be seen. He was about 35 years old and crying as I walked in the door. He was dark skinned with an accent that I was not familiar with.

I thought to myself, could this be an Ethiopian Jew as the book was still on my mind? I did not want to ask so I walked back to the chart and there it was, born in Ethiopia. I had never met an Ethiopian before and never met another again until I moved to Israel. I walked back into his room and asked, are you an Ethiopian? He said yes and that he was a Falasha. I read from the book that a Falasha is a derogatory term for a wandering Jew. I was taken aback. I asked him why he was crying and what was going on with him.

He was a diabetic and had pancreatitis. He was not allowed to eat for 6 weeks to rest his pancreas and was given IV nutrition. He was crying because this experience was reminding him of traveling in the rainforest, starving, malnourished, alone, abandoned and separated from the rest of his family.

I asked him about his plight during Operation Moses and he told me that he was airlifted with his brother to N.Y. and the rest of his family was airlifted to Israel. I then told him that he should reunite with his family in Israel. He was scared to go to Israel because the news always portrayed Israel as the dangerous hotspot in the world. I told him not to listen to the news and that once he got better he should go with his brother to his homeland – and mine.

About two months later as I was walking to the family clinic, I heard him calling my name from behind. "Dr. Gordon, I have 2 tickets to Israel for both me and my brother and I am so excited." I was so happy for him and I was so glad to be the messenger to help him reunite with his family. Yes, there are no coincidences.

CHAPTER 9

MARRIAGE AND CHILDREN

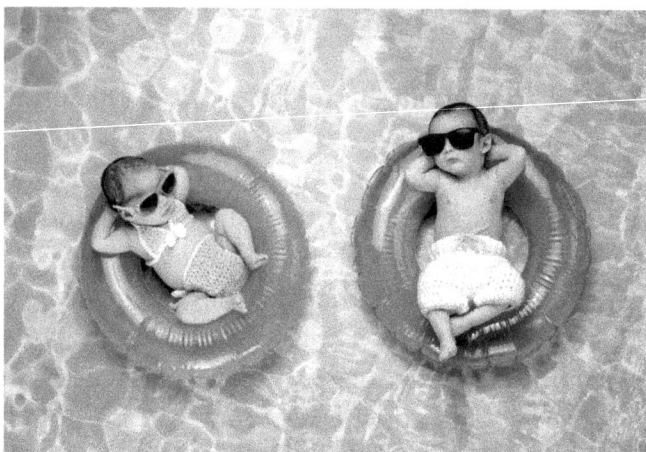

I met my husband in my third year of medical school. We had similar values as he had also studied in Israel, after not finding a meaningful purpose while living in California as a stockbroker. His father had died suddenly of pneumonia while he was in Japan teaching karate and it rattled both him and his sister enough to start searching for a more meaningful life. His sister went to Israel first and then encouraged her brother to go. Both became observant Jews. I met his sister at a women's sabbath weekend and the rest is history.

We married after six months of dating and 29 years later, have five beautiful boys. We were clueless about raising children, both of us coming from small families. I did not even know how to change a diaper, but we learned quickly, hitting some rough spots along the way.

I was pregnant within six months of marriage and gave birth in the beginning of my internship which was very challenging. We hired a live-in to help since I was working 80 plus hours a week. Our first child was very easy. I wondered why he was waking up once at night, that's how ignorant I was.

I became pregnant with my second child six months into the Internship – what was I thinking or was I? I worked long hard hours in the hospital while pregnant. My son was born with a bruise on his head and swollen eyes as if he had been in a fight. I decided after my son was born to go out into the workforce and stop my residency which was a good decision.

I now had normal hours and was not abused by the residents above me anymore. I had three jobs but was learning much more this way than in residency. I worked in walk-in clinics, as a hospitalist and at Fashion Institute of Technology in their health clinic.

Looking back at the early years, I only knew how to push myself to the very edge of my limits and really did not know how to be in the moment and enjoy life. I was programmed to be on overdrive as a former gymnast programmed to strive for perfection and fearful of financial instability as my husband was looking for work when I stopped my residency program.

If I had not been fearful, I would have nursed the baby and let my husband figure it out but at the time, the hidden fear was my driving force to keep pushing myself forward.

I was pregnant with my third child nine months after my second was born. Both my husband and I were in shock and not prepared. I continued to work through the pregnancy, but life shifted for the better as we moved to a more suburban area and into a very nice community.

I started working in a primary care practice, treating patients with osteopathic techniques. I focused on improving my osteopathic skills and taking courses and workshops across the country. I really enjoyed learning and improving my osteopathic skills and am glad I had the fortitude to "dig on" in osteopathy.

After 5 years of practicing and studying, I took my boards in Neuromuscular Medicine to become proficient in my osteopathic skills. I am blessed to be able to now teach students osteopathy at the hospitals and in my practice.

My five boys and my husband are the biggest

blessings in my life. Yes, it was twenty-nine years of hard work with its ups and downs and yes, I grew up with my boys as well.

I sometimes learned the hard way, but I got there eventually, and the hard work paid off in both the good times and rough times. I had lots of fun with my boy's – swimming, skiing, going on the trampoline while teaching them math, scuba diving, reading to them, baking and cooking with them, taking them sledding and going on various trips with them.

They were really fun boys with lots of energy, taking after both my husband and I as hyper children. It gave me such joy when they played ball together and wrestled with each other. Thank G-d we are a close family, and my husband and I would do anything for our children. We love them so much even though they can be challenging at times like most children and young adults.

I am now in a phase of my life when my children are all past the difficult teenage years. Those were hard years I must admit. Teenage years are challenging for all parents. Our children are on their own journey for the most part and as parents, we must now let them move forward to create their own lives independently of us. This process is filled with both wonder and grief.

The song, "Cat's in the Cradle," by Harry Chapin, hits home to all parents letting their children become adults. There is an empty nest feeling for all of us; for some harder than others.

I am finding more balance in my life and learning to have the wisdom to listen to my body, mind, and spirit. I am also learning how to let go daily in a conscious way.

CHAPTER 10

HOMEOPATHY

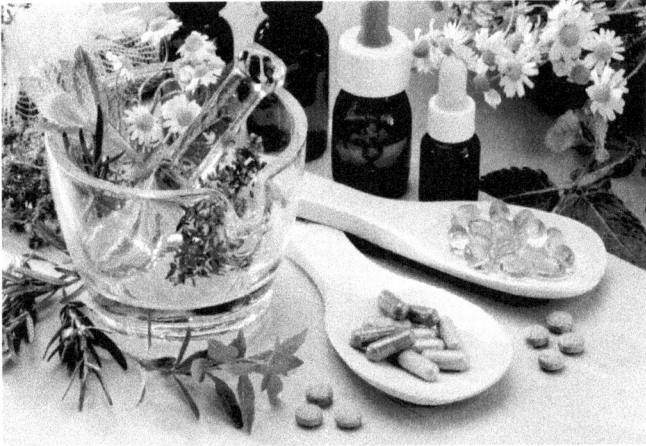

My journey towards healing through Homeopathy began in 1996. I was the director and owner of an Integrative Medical Center in N.Y. which included a classical homeopath, an acupuncturist proficient in 5 element acupuncture and Japanese acupuncture, a hypnotherapist, nutritionist, physical therapist, massage therapist and Rolfer. I would initially see patients and recommend their treatment protocol which included osteopathy.

At this point in my life, I was pregnant with my fourth child and not very happy about working so hard. I really wanted to be a mother and spend more time with my children. I was getting sick frequently, often with strep throat that did not improve with regular penicillin.

I went to see the homeopath in the practice and he prescribed a remedy that completely eliminated the strep throat. I never had strep throat again after I was given this remedy. I was very impressed.

After my fourth child was born I continued to push myself and I continued to get other infections such as viral meningitis, gastroenteritis, bronchitis, urinary tract infections but my force to keep pushing was so strong – almost unbreakable – until I was given a remedy for bronchitis which was a remedy for grief.

This was the beginning of my deep emotional pain of feeling pushed to be successful out of this incredible fear of financial instability to make something out of myself as I had grown up in a soup of financial chaos surrounded by wealthy families. I was also grieving my childhood and the feelings of being abandoned by my mother.

My husband was working in my practice and not making an independent income. I would cry desperately at night feeling from the depth of my soul helplessness, abandonment, and grief over not being nurtured myself, and my perception of not nurturing my children enough. I could not go on this way in unbearable pain. I would wake up angry at times getting only four hours of sleep at night for years after my fourth son was born.

Life was a big blur between my fourth and fifth child. I needed to feel pain and change but there seemed to be no way out but to get seriously ill.

Classical homeopathy helped me with severe chest pain coming from anxiety or anger turned inward. I took the remedy, felt angry for 3 days and then the chest pain subsided. Eventually, the last remedy I took completely took my chronic fatigue symptoms away.

I no longer had swollen glands, sore throats, or flu-like symptoms. This remedy was Nux Vomica which my homeopath told me was a good remedy for the stock broker type – pushing and then crashing.

Whenever I felt the chronic fatigue symptoms beginning to return when I overworked, I would take the remedy and the symptoms would be completely eliminated within twelve hours. I only needed to take the remedy two times and never had the symptoms again.

I learned how to pace myself and listen to myself when I felt overworked. I would meditate, simply rest, or do restorative yoga in my room. At this time of taking the remedy, my life shifted as well.

I moved to Israel with three of my sons, my husband, and father and we started a new life. I continue to commute from Israel to NY every eight weeks to work but the balance between work and enjoying life and taking care of my family is much more defined and clear for me. I was worried how I would commute eleven hours on a plane and then be strong to treat patients, but Classical Homeopathy helped me physically, emotionally, and spiritually for this transition.

Classical Homeopathy was a big player in my recovery and I am so glad that I was committed to treatment since 1996. I also receive an acupuncture treatment when I arrive in Israel to get over the jet lag and to ground myself.

Most importantly I have learned to rest for at least one day when I get off the plane and to pace myself and on occasion I have had to cancel patients at times when I feel too overworked. I have learned to say no. "No" is such an important word at times.

What is Homeopathy?

When asked about a definition of health, many people will simply say that it is the absence of disease. However, health is not just a state of being – it is a dynamic process. And the disease is individual – it is the dynamic alteration of the living whole expressed through symptoms.

In homeopathy, it is not the symptoms of a disease that are treated, but rather the living whole, because when you have a stomach ache, for example, it affects you as a whole person and not only your stomach.

By contrast, conventional medicine seeks to treat the symptoms. However, while the symptoms often disappear after treatment, the vital force does not disappear. It will find another outlet.

Healing cannot truly happen if the vital force is not healed. Homeopathy is a system of medicine that treats the vital force. Treatment seeks to complement the body's own healing energies by assisting the natural processes of the body in order to allow the body to heal itself. The person is treated as an integrated whole, taking into consideration not only the physical symptoms but also the person's mental and emotional state.

History of Homeopathy

Christian Friedrich Samuel Hahnemann (1755-1843), the founder of Homeopathy, was a German physician who became disenchanted with the medicine of his time which involved techniques such as bloodletting and purging using enemas, laxatives, and emetics.

As a linguist with knowledge of many ancient and modern languages, Hahnemann made a good deal of his living translating scientific and medical texts. In 1789 he translated the Materia Medica by William Cullen, who was one of the leading physicians of the era and first commented on the general applicability of the Law of Similars.

At one point in the book, Cullen ascribed the usefulness of Peruvian bark (cinchona) in treating malaria to its bitter and astringent properties. Hahnemann disputed Cullen's explanation in his translation, asserting that the effectiveness of Peruvian bark must derive from some other factor since he noted that there were other substances and mixtures of substances decidedly more bitter and more astringent than Peruvian bark that were not effective in treating malaria.

He then experimented by taking repeated doses of this herb until his body responded to its toxic dose exhibiting many symptoms similar to malaria. Consequently, he concluded that the reason why this herb was beneficial was because it caused symptoms similar to those of the disease it was treating. This led Hahnemann to codify the Law of Similars into a systematic medical science, marking the beginnings of a new system of medicine.

In 1810, Hahnemann published the first edition of the Organon, the book in which he explained what homeopathy is. He published five editions during his lifetime and the final, sixth, edition was published in 1921. This is the edition that is the basis for homeopathic teaching and contains 291 aphorisms in total, explaining, among others, the methodologies of case-taking, remedy selection, remedy preparation and case management.

Homeopathy was first brought to America in the mid-1800's, becoming the second most practiced healing art by public demand, until it was virtually destroyed by Big Pharma and its allies.

However, in the last 20 years, there has been a strong resurfacing of homeopathy, as it has become the fastest growing field of integrative medicine in Canada. The spring of 2007 marked a historic moment in the evolution of the Homeopathic profession in the province of Ontario. The Homeopathy Act, 2007 legislated and enacted Homeopathy as a new Regulated Health Profession in Ontario.

The Concept

At its core, homeopathy is based on the idea that each person has a vital force, a resonating frequency. This vital force is basically the energy or natural essence of the person which maintains the defense mechanism and homeostasis.

It is an energy field that integrates the mental, emotional and physical planes. If one plane is stimulated, it can affect the other two planes. Hahnemann believed that it is precisely this energy/vital force, which keeps everyone in balance.

Living matter has a fundamental mysterious

energy that makes it very different from inorganic matter. Without this vital energy, the cell, or the whole body, becomes inanimate and is dead. It is only when the vital energy is present that there is a living organism, capable of physical action and of the exercise of mental powers and ability to take hold of the spiritual forces.

The nature of energy is dynamic and penetrates every particle, every cell, every atom of the human economy. The vital force responds dynamically in health and disease.

In the simplest terms, when you are ill, according to homeopathic philosophy, your frequency changes and symptoms occur as a result of your body trying to restore you to a healthy frequency. The symptoms serve as the means by which restoration of health can be achieved. The very symptoms that allopaths suppress are the ones the body uses to get well and a homeopath surveys to find the appropriate remedy to help the body heal.

Homeopathy is, therefore, a system of medicine that treats the vital force, not symptoms – the symptoms are secondary.

The principle that like shall be cured by like, recognized by Hippocrates and Paracelsus and used by many cultures, became the basis of Hahnemann's formulation of the homeopathic doctrine: the proper remedy for a patient's disease is that substance that is capable of producing, in a healthy person, symptoms similar to those from which the patient suffers.

Remedies

Homeopathic medicines are derived from plant, mineral, or animal sources, or from healthy or diseased tissue.

Doubt about the effectiveness of the small doses is understandable, but evidence of it exists from basic science, controlled clinical studies, epidemological data, clinical outcome trials, and historical review of the field.

Homeopaths are the first to recognize that a healing response will only be initiated when a person is hypersensitive to a specific medicine. Unless the totality of symptoms experienced matches those the medicine has been found to cause when given in toxic doses, small doses of simply any medicine will not elicit therapeutic effects.

Homeopathic medicines are not only extremely diluted, they are also extremely potentized. Potentization refers to the specific process of sequential dilution with vigorous succussion.

The theory is that each consecutive dilution in conjunction with the process of succussion infiltrates the new double-distilled water and imprints upon it the fractal form of the original substance used (fractal refers to the specific consecutively smaller pattern or form within a larger pattern).

Scientific studies have shown how the information embedded in remedies spreads throughout the body (and vital force). The medicinal properties of remedies are quickly carried throughout the body water (80% of blood, 60% of the body) likely due to the electromagnetic transmission of information.

The signatures of potentized substances can even be sent electronically and transmitted into water and still work in laboratory settings.

[Benveniste, et al, Transatlantic Transfer of Digitized Antigen Signal by Telephone Link, J. Allergy Clin. Immunol. 99: S175, 1997.]

Case Taking

Besides the concept and principles mentioned above, what sets homeopathy apart from conventional, allopathic medicine is its thorough case taking technique, for which the homeopath takes a minimum of two hours at the time of the initial visit.

While homeopathy treats the vital force rather than the symptoms, it is still crucial that the homeopath has a thorough knowledge of the symptomatology from a medical point of view in order not to confuse the symptoms of the disease with that characteristic of the patient.

Only the more characteristic information from

the patient which is not relevant to the disease will lead to the curative remedy. For example, asking questions like it feels better with warm drinks, better with movement, better at night, agitated, fearful, sweats easily... all related to the nature of the person and their presentation while sick.

It is the symptoms from the source of the inner self, unrelated to pathology, that are of utmost importance.

As such, through its deep case taking and corrsponding selection of a remedy which encompasses the totality of symptoms, homeopathy, unlike any other modality (with the exception of acupuncture, cranial therapy and energy healing), treats patients at the deepest possible level, affecting cures not only at the physical but at the mental and emotional levels too.

Widespread Usage of Homeopathy

In many countries around the world, the homeopathic system of medicine is considered a respected alternative to allopathy and in India, it is a regulated system equal to allopathy. In an excerpt from an article in the New India Press, dated December 24, 2005, titled, "WHO Recognition for Homeopathy" the worldview on homeopathy is discussed as follows:

"Deviating from the trend of rejecting homeopathy treatment and medicine as mere placebos, the

World Health Organization (WHO) has declared that homeopathy is the second most used medical system internationally. 'Clinical trials have proved that this method of treatment has been successful."

Homeopathy has found widespread support in all walks of life:

Famous Quotes:

"..[Homeopathy] cures a larger percentage of cases than any other method of treatment and is beyond all doubt safer, more economical, and the most complete medical science."

~ Mahatma Gandhi
(Homeopathy is now the most popular form of medicine in India.)

"...[Homeopathy is a].. progressive and aggressive step in medicine."

~ John D Rockefeller

"....You may honestly feel grateful that homeopathy survived the attempts of the [orthodox physicians] to destroy it."

~ Mark Twain (author), Harper's Magazine, February 1890.

More recently, the following have also endorsed Homeopathic Medicine:

The entire British Royal family, including Her

Majesty Queen Elizabeth II and His Royal Highness, Prince Charles, the Prince of Wales.

"Homeopathy is a highly developed health practice that uses a systematic approach to the totality of a person's health. Anyone seeking a fuller understanding of health and healing will find Homeopathy extremely important and applicable."

~ Gay Gaer Luce. Ph.D.,
(science writer; twice winner of the national science writer's award)

By adopting a worldview derived from complex systems theory in which the whole equals more than the sum of its parts, a new perspective for medicine and health care emerges.

The science and art of homeopathy embody what many people envision as a 21st-century medicine. It is a medical approach that respects the wisdom of the body. It utilizes medicines that stimulate the body's own immune and defense system to initiate the healing process.

In a sense, the role of homeopathic remedies is similar to that of enzymes and hormones in controlling homeostatic balance within the organism to maintain a functioning harmony between all parts. Thus, the minute doses of homeopathic potencies act as a catalyst to stimulate the body's natural defense mechanism.

Homeopathic medicines are individualized according to the totality of the person's physical, emotional, and mental symptoms. While this medical approach is widely recognized to be safe, it can also be potentially very effective in treating the new types of diseases that are afflicting us now and will affect us in the 21st century.

CHAPTER 11

ACUPUNCTURE

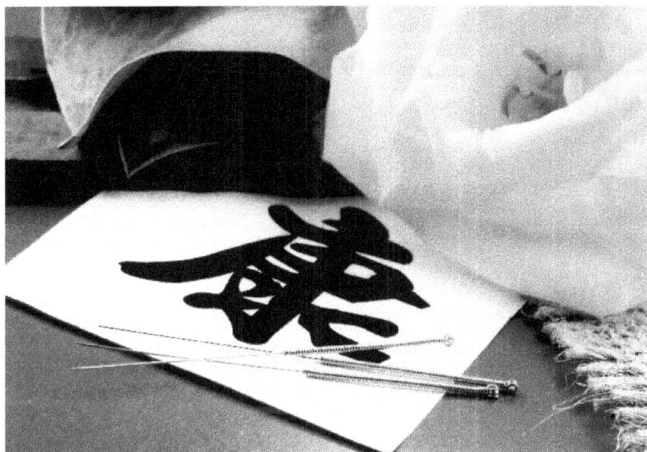

What Is Five Element Acupuncture?

I am often asked about Five-Element acupuncture, which is the classical form of Chinese medicine. According to the principles of Chinese Medicine, all change – in the universe and in your body – occurs in five distinct stages.

Each of these stages is associated with a particular time of year, a specific element in nature, and a pair of organs in the body. Change links together the seasons of the year, aspects of nature, and your body's organs and bodily processes.

A practitioner of classical acupuncture uses this principle to diagnose and treat health problems, linking specific foods, herbs, and acupuncture points to the restoration of your vital energy.

According to classical Chinese medicine – Fire, Earth, Metal, Water & Wood – are elements that exist in all living things. When an imbalance occurs, illness can result. Five-Element diagnosis and treats the element that is out of balance, enabling healing to occur in the body, mind and spirit.

Each element has an odor, color, sound and emotion attached to it that can be perceived when that element is out of balance. In addition, each patient's unique body, mind and spirit are taken into account when determining diagnosis and treatment, so that each individual receives customized treatment.

Each person has a unique balance of the five elements – so no two people are the same, regardless of the similarity of their symptoms.

The goal of a Five Element practice is to pinpoint and treat the underlying causative factor of "dis-ease". Treating the causative factor enables the person to heal completely.

This is the essential difference between acupuncture and western (or allopathic) medicine, where patients presenting the same symptoms are usually treated in the exact same way and given the exact same dose of the exact same prescription drug.

An acupuncture patient typically receives 90 minutes of time during an initial intake session – to diagnose and treat an imbalance and, in most cases, feels markedly better even after the first treatment, as healing begins.

This is one reason why more people are turning to acupuncture treatments – for individualized care, a personal relationship with the practitioner, natural treatment free from adverse side effects and the promotion of improved sleep and overall calmative effect.

Five Elements to Health

The model of the Five Elements, handed down from ancient China, is both the foundation for a system of medicine and a symbolic representation that provides a way "to live the fullest life." The elements are essentially universal archetypes that can guide us in the art of living.

One of the great joys about being knowledgeable in classical acupuncture is that it teaches us so much about ourselves and about nature. It actually brings us closer to nature, closer to the real joy in life; and it give us a sense of proportion. Thus, we enrich our lives by understanding our bodies, minds and spirits according to the laws of nature.

J.R. Worsley, my sister's mentor who reintroduced Five Element Constitutional Acupuncture to the west, emphasized nourishing the *underlying imbalance via treatment of the CF ('Causative Factor') or Constitutional Factor and said, "this system of medicine is based on the most solid foundation of any system of medicine in the world. It is wholly based on natural laws. Man cannot pollute it; man cannot change it; man cannot improve upon it."

The aim of Classical Five Element Acupuncture is to isolate the cause of disease. Treating symptoms does not address the root cause of an imbalance. A symptom is seen as a distress signal coming from the body or the mind or the spirit, crying out for help. It is not the cause. The symptom acts as a warning, alerting us to a deeper underlying cause that must be addressed.

What is striking is how treatment focused on the CF has the ability to initiate extraordinary changes in a person's health and sense of well-being. As the CF is the primary imbalance, change is commonly initiated in other organs and elements not treated directly. This is due to the relationships between the elements expressed in the sheng (creative) and ke (controlling) cycles.

My sister, my closest friend and our family acupuncturist, has gotten my family out of many crises throughout the years. She once helped my husband when he was acutely ill with a severe stomach virus that caught him off guard. He was vomiting nonstop for which I tried using intravenous medication to no avail.

My sister was working that day in my office and happened to walk upstairs to see my husband with an IV in his arm keeling over. I was about to bring him to the emergency room. She treated him with five element acupuncture and his symptoms completely resolved within thirty minutes. She has helped our family time and again.

I have two sons with allergies and asthma and both were treated successfully with acupuncture. I have a son who had suffered from middle ear infections starting when he was two months old. Acupuncture helped with his fevers and pain. There was one instance where he was treated for fever and within two minutes the fever went from 102° to 98.6°F, right in front of our eyes.

The pediatrician wanted to start him on antibiotics, but my gut feeling was that his system was very weak because I had been on antibiotics three times while I was pregnant. I wanted to build and strengthen his immune system. We did get him completely symptom- free of ear infections within six months without antibiotics.

I remember one time I had a tooth extraction and I had anesthesia after the extraction. I suffered from insomnia and irregular uterine bleeding. My sister gave me one treatment and both insomnia and the bleeding completely subsided.

My father always requested acupuncture treatments from my sister as it would help his leg cramps from varicose veins as well as arthritic pain in his hands.

Acupuncture was very useful for my mother in the course of her illness with Chronic Lymphocytic Leukemia (CLL). It would help with increasing my mother's energy and appetite.

In the last hours of my mother's life, my sister treated her with acupuncture using spirit points to help her "let go" as my mother had such a hard time with the thought of leaving this world.

I also treated my mother with Cranial Therapy and within two hours of both treatments she had her hands over her heart resting comfortably and peacefully. She opened her eyes one last time and looked at us by her bedside as we said our goodbyes. She then took one more breath and was gone.

Over the years, time and again, I have seen my sister use her magic hands and change people's lives physically, emotionally and spiritually.

Today acupuncture is an accepted modality of treatment and many insurance companies will pay for treatments.

I wholeheartedly recommend acupuncture for

hormone imbalances, pain, insomnia, post anesthesia, allergies, asthma, bronchitis, sinus infections, ear infections, acne and pretty much any imbalance. I also recommend that everyone have an acupuncture treatment when there's a change of season to adapt to the environmental change on all levels.

The case histories that follow are from my sister, Sharon's patients that were seen in our office. These case histories will show you just how powerful acupuncture can be as a healing modality.

Acupuncture Helps Gynecological Imbalances

The Case of Uncontrolled Menstrual Bleeding

A peri-menopausal woman had hemorrhagic bleeding during her periods.

The excessive menstrual bleeding every month lead to anemia. The patient felt bad physically and was nervous because she never knew what was going to happen. The excessive bleeding completely changed her lifestyle. She didn't want to go on vacation or even out because she did not know when she would bleed heavily and would have to stay at home due to this condition.

She was a school teacher and her gynecologist didn't know how she was able to work. There were times she bled so heavily, had clots and she became anemic as a result. They were frightening experiences for her and after these bouts, she felt fatigued and so ill that she missed work and was in bed for ten days taking large doses of Iron.

Finally, her doctor put her on synthetic progesterone. She was on the hormone for two weeks and then off for two weeks. When she tried this, within six hours of not taking the hormone her hemorrhagic bleeding began anew.

She remained on the synthetic progesterone for two years until a routine blood test revealed she had elevated liver enzymes. The gynecologist told her to immediately stop taking the hormone and recommended a hysterectomy as her only option.

She consulted with Dr. Barbara Gordon-Cohen who recommended trying acupuncture. With much skepticism, she began acupuncture treatments once a week while gradually reducing the synthetic progesterone. She no longer experienced heavy bleeding and within eight weeks was completely off the synthetic hormone.

The patient stated, "Whereas the hemorrhagic bleeding changed my whole lifestyle, the success of the acupuncture also changed everything for mc – back to a healthy and happy lifestyle. I do not understand how the acupuncture works but the whole experience has been very relaxing and needless to say very rewarding."

In Chinese medicine, the Spleen is responsible for holding the blood in the vessels. Uncontrollable menstrual bleeding can be viewed as an imbalance in the Spleen Official or Spleen Qi deficiency. The Liver Official responsible for storing the blood was also imbalanced.

Acupuncture supports the Qi of ALL the

Officials in the body that helped resolve hemorrhagic bleeding.

Acupuncture Helps Boost the Immune System

Acupuncture is an excellent alternative to over-the-counter allergy medications and it comes with no side effects like drowsiness or dryness. Acupuncture is noted for its ability to strengthen the immune system. How does it do this? Using acupuncture points along the meridian pathways stimulates the release of specific neurotransmitters, that, in turn, affects immune system function.

The Case of Severe Allergic Reaction

A 35-year-old mother with an 8-month-old was exposed to mold during a vacation at a beachfront resort. The mold spores in the unit she was staying caused non-stop sneezing, itchy eyes, ears, nose, and throat. She was just about to take allergy medication when I treated her on her underlying cause reflected in the five elements which for her was the Wood element.

The Liver and Gallbladder points calmed her allergic response within about thirty minutes. I treated her again the next day to fortify her Liver Qi and the sneezing, watery eyes and itchy throat symptoms all resolved. She did not need to take an antihistamine and was very impressed by the treatment results.

The Case of Antibiotics Weakening the Immune System

A 27-year-old woman who had been treated for Clostridium difficile, often called C. difficile, is a bacterium that can cause symptoms ranging from diarrhea to life-threatening inflammation of the colon, came to me after months of taking antibiotics. Her immune system was compromised by the strong antibiotic and its long-term use that resolved her C. difficile.

She was extremely fatigued, developed a severe case of acne and became sensitive to dairy products.

I treated her over 12 weeks and in that time, was able to resolve the acne and strengthen her immune system. I used moxibustion on the immune strengthening points on her back and limbs and – within the first two treatments, I could see a marked improvement in her energy.

Moxibustion is a way to therapeutically apply direct heat onto an acupuncture point in the form of a cone that is derived from mugwort, an herb known for its ability to burn evenly.

Acupuncture Helps Fight Off the Common Cold

I once told a patient to see me for treatment within the first 24-36 hours coming down with common cold symptoms. When she began to get chills and fever she came in and I treated her. The next time I saw the patient, she reported that after treatment all her symptoms had been exacerbated. She went through the entire cycle of her virus within only twenty-four hours.

Acupuncture Helps Postoperative Recovery

The Case of the Severely Depressed Patient Following Knee Surgery

---

I often tell patients that acupuncture speeds up the healing process following surgery. Many people suffer from the after effects of having been anesthetized. Depending on how long the surgery is, anesthesia can affect everything from your energy, to your digestion, to your moods.

An 88-year-old woman came to me following knee surgery on the advice of her daughter who I had been treating for some time.

The daughter said that her mother's surgery was a success but that she was extremely fatigued and was severely depressed. So much so, the doctors put her on antidepressants. She was also extremely fearful and had cold hands and feet.

My first treatment was a detox treatment that revealed her heart Qi was affected by the operation. As we age, our Kidney Qi is affected, and the operation additionally depleted the kidney energy as well. I fortified both heart and kidney energies.

Once these were balanced the patient came out of her depression and was able to stop the antidepressants. I only needed to see her two times for a complete recovery.

Acupuncture to The Rescue in a Crisis

The Case of the Doctor with a Husband/Wife Block

Acupuncturists take many pulses along the radial artery during treatment to assess what is going on in the body's energy channels. There are three pulse positions on both the left and right wrists of the patient along the radial artery at the superficial, middle and deep levels of the pulse. Practitioners use their pointer, middle and ring fingers to take pulses on both wrists throughout the treatment.

Acupuncturists use their pulse taking skills to get a complete pulse picture. Where blocks between the pulses are found, they are treated to allow the pulses to return to balance.

In Five Element Acupuncture, the most serious of all the blocks is called a husband/wife block: all the pulses on the left (husband) side are much weaker than all the pulses on the right (wife) side. A husband/wife block, if left untreated, can result in a downward spiral of the patient leading to death.

I found a husband/wife block on Dr. Barbara after she had flown to Las Vegas from NY to take an eight-hour family practice board examination. At the time, she was nursing a six-month-old baby, raising four additional sons, all while her multi-modality practice in New York was going through an upheaval. Dr. Barbara was extremely fatigued with this additional stress along with working long hours. By the time she got to sit for her boards she had used up all her energy reserves.

After taking the eight-hour exam,

she was even more fatigued and awoke in the middle of the night with anxiety. She said she felt like she was going into a dark tunnel and was going to literally die. Her pulses revealed a husband/wife block which I treated. The acupuncture treatment resurrected her and brought her out of that dark tunnel immediately.

CHAPTER 12

MORE HOMEOPATHY CASES

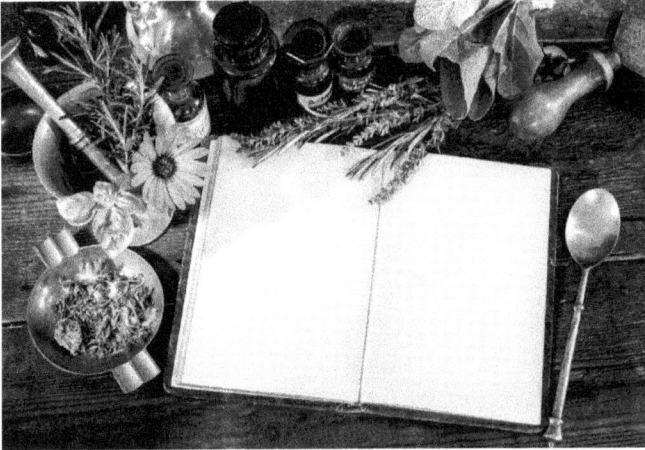

There are many instances when I have referred cases to a classical homeopath. I remember two times when after taking a health history, I called a homeopath into the room.

In the first case, of a mother and daughter, the daughter was complaining of having a chronic cough for a year without relief from inhalers, antibiotics, and antacids. She said she came to me as a last-

ditch effort as she was desperate to get better.

I saw them quarreling in the office and had a feeling that there was a strong emotional component related to this case. I called the homeopath in and he told me that he would hope to have success with this patient.

I asked detailed questions about her cough, her preferences of food, environment, habits, hobbies, activity, relationships and very detailed questions about her relationship with her parents. Her mother had just gotten divorced and she was overbearing towards her daughter.

The classical homeopath gave her a remedy after thoroughly reviewing her case. Her cough subsided within the first week of taking the remedy.

Another case involved an infant with a pertussis infection. She was coughing non-stop until she turned blue. The cough was dry and hacking and worse at night. She was a clingy type of baby with a sweet disposition. The homeopath gave her a remedy which completely alleviated the cough. The mother was thrilled.

I've had many cases of intestinal bacterial infections (gastroenteritis) with giardia, and C.Difficile in which antibiotics only gave temporary relief and then recurred.

I referred them to a classical homeopath in each case and diarrhea and abdominal pain completely subsided within a week's time and never returned. I have also seen good results in ridding pinworms in children.

I have seen success with pain from rheumatoid arthritis and sprains as well. I clearly remember one case where the child had poison ivy with a huge blister on the palm of his right hand. The mother refused to have her son go on steroids for the inflammation.

The homeopath in the office gave her Rhus tox which is poison ivy, in a very diluted dose of 200 c. The very next day the blister completely resolved. I have to say I was surprised. I thought she would need steroids, but I was wrong.

CHAPTER 13

NATURAL HORMONE THERAPY

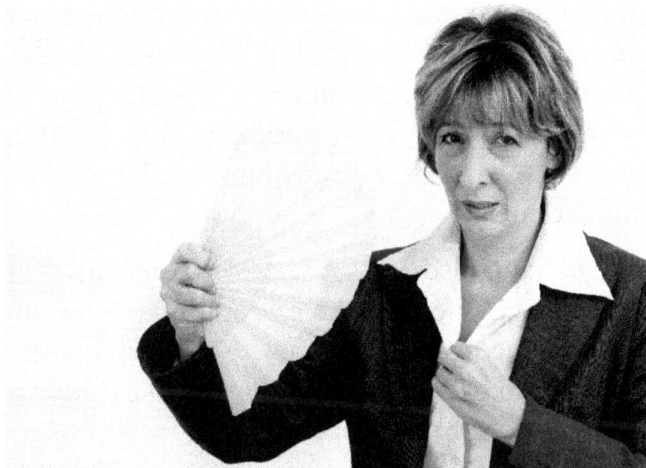

I got involved with bioidentical hormones (natural hormones), even though I never learned about them in medical school when I started working for Dr. Michael Schachter, M.D. in 1992.

I was introduced to the use of them for women who had menopausal symptoms such as hot flashes, insomnia, anxiety, chest pain, dry skin, vaginal dryness/pain and hair loss. I also learned about the symptoms of low testosterone in both men and women experiencing fatigue, irritability, low sex drive or no sex drive. DHEA (dehydroepiandrosterone), which is a precursor

DR. BARBARA GORDON-COHEN, D.O.

to estrogen and testosterone, is found to be a vitality hormone. DHEA may help with sex drive, energy, and also may prevent heart disease and osteoporosis. As we age, this hormone declines.

DHEA modulates endothelial function, reduces inflammation, improves insulin sensitivity, blood flow, cellular immunity, body composition, bone metabolism, sexual function, and physical strength in frailty and provides neuroprotection, improves cognitive function, and memory enhancement.

I had attended an A.C.A.M. conference in Anaheim California (American College for the Advancement of Medicine) where I had the privilege to hear prominent doctors in the field of natural hormone replacement therapy on the cutting edge.

I met with one doctor who introduced me to using natural long acting T3 for people who suffered from underactive thyroid symptoms but who had normal lab tests or the synthetic thyroid hormones they were taking were not resolving their symptoms.

These symptoms included: fatigue, dry skin, hair loss, chipping nails, intolerance to cold and always feeling cold, muscle aches, depression, poor healing, easy bruisability, weight gain, and difficulty becoming pregnant.

I also learned about the Dr. Broda Barnes

protocol using natural desiccated armor thyroid or nature-throid. Not only did these patients have these symptoms they also had low body temperatures.

According to the Broda Barnes Protocol, one places an oral glass thermometer under the armpit for 10 minutes upon awakening while still in bed and the basal body temperature should read between 97.8 and 98. 2. It is most accurate during the menses (period). The temperature reading would help determine if a patient was a candidate for using thyroid hormone therapy.

The other protocol from the book, Wilson's Syndrome, using long-acting T3 resets thyroid function and eliminates the production of reverse T3.

I found out inactive T3 was produced when one was under stress and more predominant among the Irish and American Indian populations probably because they suffered from a history of famines which caused their thyroid gland to slow down to compensate for lack of food and to increase survival.

This underactive thyroid state was then passed down genetically. The temperatures for this protocol were taken under the tongue three times a day using a regular glass oral thermometer and the normal temperature was 98.6.

All of the patients that I encountered who had

symptoms of underactive thyroid all had low body temperatures and the goal was to restore body temperatures to normal levels thus resolving symptoms.

The key to restoring the temperatures also laid in the function of the adrenal glands. The adrenal glands are the foundation to treating thyroid dysfunction. The use of adrenal glandulars and/or herbs such as ashwagandha and magnolia, acupuncture, massage, reflexology, osteopathy, meditation, yin yoga or restorative yoga helps balance the adrenals to create a more efficient environment for the thyroid to stop producing reverse T3 and start producing T3: the active thyroid hormone.

I started to treat people with hypometabolic state or thyroid dysfunction according to their symptoms, lab results and body temperatures and I had much success with these patients.

One patient who switched from Synthroid to Armour thyroid was able to get pregnant and maintained her pregnancy after more than two years of trying to get pregnant taking Synthroid. I had many patients rid themselves of their sluggish thyroid symptoms either using Armour thyroid, Naturethroid or long acting T3.

They now felt warmer, had more energy, had stronger nails and decreased hair loss, lost weight, had more motivation and got their lives back. I realize this whole natural hormone replacement therapy is an art as well as a science.

Listening for the patient's history, stressors, habits and lifestyle are keys to helping uncover what will heal them. Certain lab tests are ordered and sometimes saliva tests are ordered to check hormone levels and adjust according to symptoms, labs and body temperatures for thyroid patients.

They now call this whole process "Functional Medicine." Back in 1991, they called it Integrative Medicine and then Complementary Medicine. I was naturally very inclined to follow this path, seeing the limitations of conventional medicine and wanting to help as many people as I could.

After all, that was my calling – to be a doctor that heals.

I would plow through as many books as I could when my children were asleep and learn as much as I could from my mentors.

Natural hormone replacement hit home for me after I had my fifth child. I was so low in both estrogen and progesterone (remember I was a gymnast for twelve years with very low body fat so I was already depleted in hormones prior to having children) that I had hot flashes while sleeping, and severe chest pain and PMS for two weeks prior to my menses.

I was my own experiment. I first used natural

progesterone which helped my PMS symptoms such as insomnia, anxiety and chest pain. Then I started taking low doses of mostly estriol creme which helped completely resolve my chest pain as well as the hot flashes.

I had seen a psychopharmacologist prior for these symptoms because I was so desperate to get rid of the constant chest pain. He gave me a low dose of Risperdal, an antipsychotic medication which used in low doses helps with anxiety. I took half the lowest dose which alleviated the chest pain, but I could not get my body out of bed. That was the end of that path.

I once had a patient tell me that her doctor prescribed Neurontin and Effexor for hot flashes and insomnia. She told me the doctor discouraged synthetic hormones because they could cause cardiovascular disease or stroke and told her that the antidepressants and Neurontin would help her.

She still had the hot flashes and she gained 30 pounds. She was miserable, especially about her weight gain.

I thought to myself – how sad is that. These doctors don't know about natural hormones and the drug companies do not dispense them because they are not allowed to patent anything that is completely natural.

This patient eventually went off the antidepressants and was prescribed an estrogen hormone patch and had since lost most of her original weight gain. I would have put her on natural hormone replacement of both estrogen and progesterone in its natural form which would mimic the body's hormone production before menopause.

I would use more estriol than estradiol as estriol has been reported to have less carcinogenic effects than estradiol and is not metabolized by the liver. I use on average 80% estriol and 20% estradiol to treat menopausal symptoms rather than 100% estradiol.

There have been studies done on natural hormones but not large studies due to a lack of proper funding.

If you think about it, the synthetic hormones that our cells are not used to may have side effects even at low doses. The natural hormones are so easy to work with and the side effects are only from giving too much so this is where the art of prescribing comes in.

I feel so blessed to have turned the lives of many men and women around with natural hormones. They once had some or all of the symptoms including fatigue, depression, hot flashes, insomnia, anxiety, overweight, cold, dry skin, hair loss, poor wound healing, easy bruisability, frequent infections and chest pain and are now thriving and feeling great.

I have been working with natural hormones since 1992 and in those twenty-five years, I have had two cases of breast cancer. One was hormone receptor negative meaning that it was not related to hormones. I would say over the course of 24 years I have had an over 90% success rate.

Doctors are now starting to learn about bioidentical hormones but some for the wrong reasons. They are burnt out with the insurance system and are scrambling at another platform of medicine that does not require insurance.

The bioidentical courses online are advertising to doctors that this could be their ticket out of being stuck in the conventional system's dependency on insurance companies.

The doctors are now victims of these insurance companies that tell them what drugs they can and can't prescribe, audit notes and are not paying the doctor for some bogus reason. Doctors are now desperate to get out of the insurance companies stranglehold
on them.

I am again blessed to have made the decision for the right reasons and to have followed my beliefs and my gut about healing at a young age. I am glad that I was not manipulated by the system like so many of my colleagues. I was very idealistic and wanted to genuinely help people and did not go into medicine for the money.

The hard work paid off and my patients are very appreciative of their improved quality of life. I have seen life changing results and feel deeply satisfied with my profession.

PART TWO

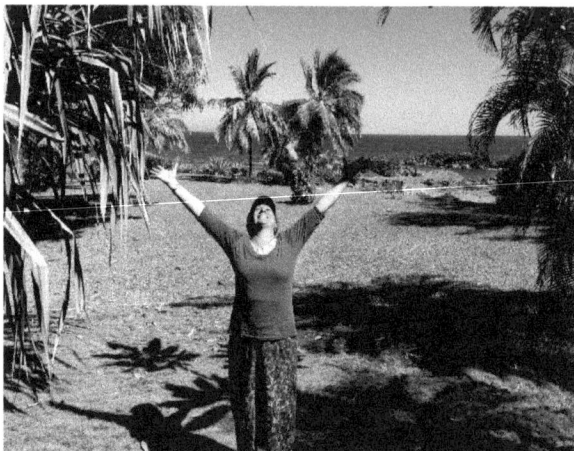

CHAPTER 14

TAPPING INTO THE UNCONSCIOUS MIND

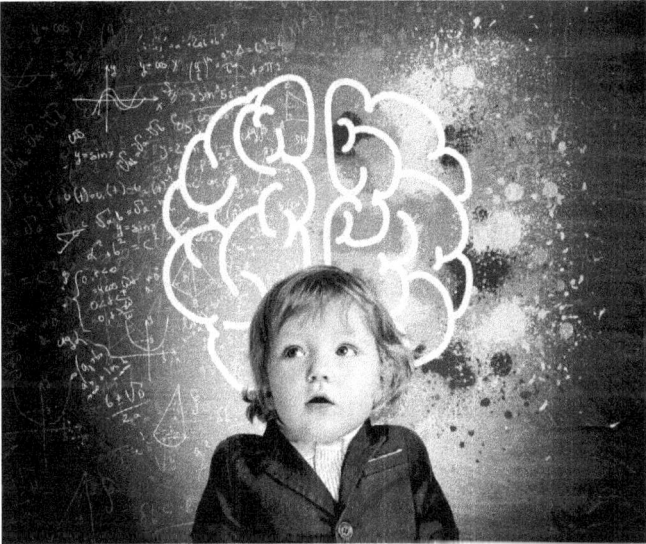

The modalities in this chapter can assist in tapping into your unconscious mind which represents memories that you are not aware of consciously. (One should not choose modalities of treatments, if mentally unstable, without the support of a qualified therapist).

My own personal journey with my unconscious mind initially began when I "hit the wall" and all my repressed childhood wounds started to resurface.

After my fifth and last child was born, I started working with a hypnotherapist who would guide me into a deep state of relaxation and then have me go back in time. I visually saw myself at about 4 years old and completely alone, feeling abandoned by my mother. I had nowhere to turn and I felt so vulnerable.

I started to cry in the session from my heart as I felt the pain of the experience that I never really felt growing up. My mother worked full-time from the time I was two and a half years old. I had been in various playgroups, and with babysitters.

While all my experiences were good, I was very aware that when my mother was home with me she was not really there. She was mostly on the phone with her friends or self-absorbed. She could not handle my emotional or physical pain as a child.

She had no tolerance and later on when I started to do **The Journey**™, (Developed by Brandon Bays), with a facilitator, I realized she was incapable of dealing with my pain.

I remember when I was in kindergarten the teacher asked us if anyone had a dream they would like to share with the class. I raised my hand. I told them of a recent dream about my mother abandoning me in a drug store as she left me to go home. I was crying because in the dream I could not find my mother and I was scared.

My mother worked for a pharmaceutical company and I guess I felt like she left me all the time to go to her work. I would take taxis from kindergarten to my babysitter daily. The babysitter also took care of foster children in her home. I really enjoyed going there as I had many children to play with and the mother was like a grandma who fed us delicious Italian food.

I often did not want to go home when my mom came to pick me up. My mother yelled a lot and it scared me and made me feel like I was walking on eggshells. I developed a pattern of keeping my feelings inside.

It was a great release to uncover the repressed feelings of being alone, but it took a long time to move forward from the feeling of abandonment. It expressed itself in different ways that I began to understand as I went to cognitive and psychoanalytic therapy.

I remember one instance going shopping for food alone. I left my children with my husband and I experienced palpitations as I felt the rawness of abandoning my own children and flashbacks of my mom leaving me. Hypnotherapy allowed me to feel the pain in my body and tap into what was going on emotionally under that pain.

At one point when I was in my office, I had severe pain in my forearms. This occurred after I had moved a huge practice to another building down the street after one of the practitioners stole patients from me and started his own practice on the same floor.

I worked with this man for five years and referred many patients to him and then he betrayed me. My anger towards him turned inward and it started to manifest as pain.

After moving all the files, desks, equipment, supplements, and getting the new practice established, the severe pain in my forearms surfaced. I was so desperate to relieve the pain that I took lidocaine and injected the trigger points in both forearms.

At that moment I felt so deeply the feeling of being alone as a child and as an adult. I felt so alone with no one there to help me. I cried my eyes out as the emotional pain flooded out of me. It was stored at a cellular level for all those years and now I was opening a closed wound. Little did I know that the trigger point injections would do this to me.

I just thought that the injections would help my physical pain. I tried taking a muscle relaxant one time and it took the physical pain away but immediately created emotional pain which I have to say is worse than physical pain, so I never tried another muscle relaxant again.

The process of coming to terms with abandonment in the past took several years and I did succeed. I also succeeded in gaining my own voice and self-confidence. I think that being pushed away by my mother and hearing her yell left me without a voice to speak up for myself.

May my mom rest in peace. She also had great qualities: she was affectionate, fun, supportive of all my interests, and her love for me knew no bounds. I know she did her very best as a mom and really, we all do as mothers with whatever limitations we have. I am sure my children will have their complaints too as this is the cycle of life.

Did you know that cellular memory, unlike brain memory, actually stores experiences not just facts and figures? Experiences tend to be stored as impressions and are viewed from all the senses, not just visual.

For example, the brain retrieves a memory and will most likely show you a picture or a list or a graphic. Cells retrieve a memory and will give you a body sensation such as pain or tension or tingling or you may be 'frozen with fear'. You may also sense a fragrance, taste, sounds or any combination of senses that held the imprint of the experience.

Cellular memory can store memories of physical trauma like accidents, cuts, bruises, surgeries, or abuse; emotional trauma like heartache, fear, guilt and anger; and mental trauma that manifests in low self-esteem, unworthiness, worry, etc. When trauma is suppressed into the cellular memory, that energy can get stuck.

Not everyone agrees that cellular memory exists. Scientists doubt it because there isn't a way to effectively measure it. Unlike brain waves and stimulation, cellular memory occurs in all cells, and there's no proof that the memory is actually stored there.

But some researchers are beginning to share ideas that support cellular memory. Think back to the basic conditioned response as developed and observed by Ivan Pavlov, the Russian physiologist best known for his work in classical conditioning. Ringing a bell produced salivation when paired with food initially. Thereafter, salivation happened with only the bell for association. A body response, a sensory response, a muscle memory response to an event.

Post-traumatic stress syndrome (PTSD) also relates to cellular memory. Survivors of stress or trauma exhibit multiple signs of ongoing memory in their bodies through physical symptoms such as shaking, an inability to move or act and sweating. Emotional symptoms such as sadness, fear or anger. Mental symptoms such as aggression, the inability to make decisions and powerlessness.

Unfortunately, there are many situations in which it is not safe to experience suppressed trauma.

This can occur when the trauma was too overwhelming to be experienced and it will thus be too overwhelming to re-experience.

It can also occur when the trauma is ongoing and there is never a "safe time or place" to release it.

It is easy to see how this can occur in extreme situations like acts of violence, abuse, or even near-death experiences. It can also, however, occur in situations that do not seem as extreme such as trauma suppressed into their cellular memory resulting from their experience of being adopted, the death of a loved one, moving from a childhood home to a new home, emotional abuse, physical abuse, neglect, and many other experiences. In these situations, the energy of the trauma becomes stuck and remains suppressed into the cellular memory.

The problem with suppressed cellular memory is not only does it limit our ability to live freely and joyfully, but it can also support the body in developing a physical illness.

CHAPTER 15

THE JOURNEY™

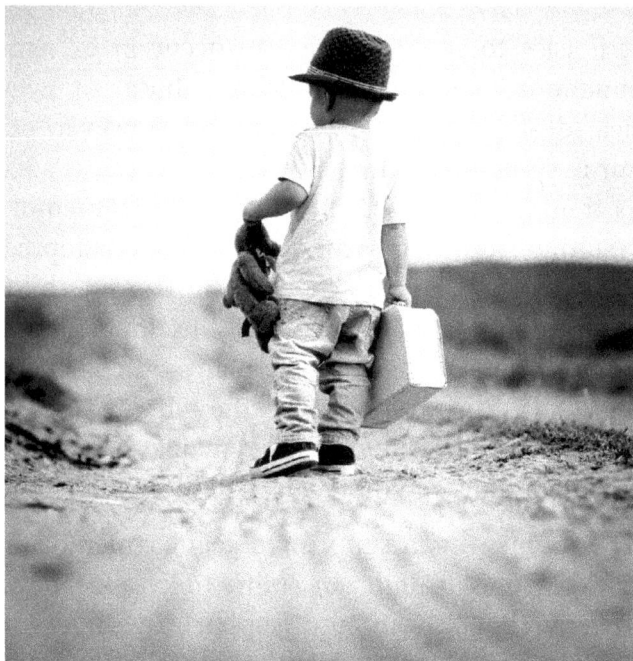

The Journey™ work began for me after a patient told me of her experience with it and how it helped her release emotional trauma as well as uncover layers of anger, fear, and grief.

Ultimately, she said she came to a place of genuine forgiveness of others who caused her emotional pain.

She told me to read the book, The Journey™ by Brandon Bays. This work is globally recognized and a critically acclaimed healing and transformational modality to uncover and awaken your limitless potential, and to apply it in every area of your life.

This simple, yet powerful step-by-step method of overcoming a wide variety of challenges, from physical ailments to emotional issues or shut down, in relationship problems and with career or performance issues.

Brandon Bays, the founder of The Journey™ work, is an internationally acclaimed speaker, best-selling author, and mind-body healing expert.

In 1992, Bays was diagnosed with a basketball-sized tumor. Because of her background and strong belief system around holistic healing, she put all of it (nutrition, herbology, kinesiology, meditation and guided introspection) into a carefully planned natural healing regimen. Both she and her doctors were amazed that within only 6 1/2 weeks, she was completely healed with no drugs, no surgery, and no pain.

Inspired by the studies of famed endocrinologist Deepak Chopra and renowned cellular biologist Dr. Candace Pert, The Journey™ developed its own unique approach to awakening and cellular healing and has become a potent blend of cutting-edge tools to access the true human potential that knows no bounds.

After reading this book, I had my husband do the exercises in the back of the book with me. I was lying down and my husband followed the guide, putting me into a relaxed state by having me relax each body part until I was completely relaxed.

What came up for me was my experience as a teenager when my sister came home from college deeply depressed. I could not communicate with her as she was completely shut down. My parents did not communicate with me about what was going on with my sister, so I was left out in the dark. I did not know at the time how to react, but I was scared and alone in my feelings.

My mechanism to deal with stress was to tune it out, study and be productive. I found myself sobbing in front of my husband feeling the pain of seeing my sister so depressed and lifeless. Two hours had gone by as I emotionally unraveled the suppressed pain.

I then sought out a Journey™ facilitator recommended by a patient and had her come to my home for three hours of Journey™ work. I was really impressed by the emotional work that we did. First, she had me relax every body part and then we went back into my past to my relationship with my mother as she was the one that I had issues with unconsciously.

I saw myself as a 6-year-old girl, very alone with nowhere to turn for emotional or physical support. I felt angry and my body began to experience a burning sensation all over.

The instructor had me imagine that I was sitting by a campfire and that a close mentor was by my side to support me. She had me go back to my mother's youth and what my mother's challenges had been. She had a controlling father who did not let her be a child. I felt for her that she was so confined as a child.

We then looked at the relationship of my grandmother and grandfather and I thought that my grandmother should have divorced him as he was a tyrant and so controlling of his children and my grandmother. I was truly able to forgive my mother with all my heart as she had her limitations from her past.

I then felt this incredible feeling of connectedness to all my family and to G-d that we are all one. I felt this beautiful white light over me and at complete peace.

That night I had a dream that many friends of mine were taking advantage of me for prescription medications. I realized that as a young girl I learned to not have a voice as I was scared of my mother's yelling. I avoided confrontation because my mother was so good at confronting others, to the point of my feeling embarrassed and wanting to hide in a corner.

The next day I called the friends that were asking me for prescriptions and told them I could not do them any more favors and that they should see their doctor. This was the first time I felt empowered and from there I started using my voice but in a calm way.

This session helped me so much that I was able to nurture my mother completely and with love toward the end of her life when she was dying from Leukemia. She stayed in my home and I took care of her along with my family and sister until her last breath.

She rejected nurturing from us in the beginning because she might not have been nurtured herself. She somehow felt bad that I had to help her. I told her how grateful I felt to take care of her and that it gave me pleasure to be there for her. She was so grateful to me and so appreciative of my family for helping her in her final days.

My mother rarely discussed her childhood and if she did it was with trepidation. She never really worked through her issues as a child as many of our parents had nowhere to turn or did not believe in therapy. My mother definitely was one to suppress her feelings and maybe this is what caused her illness.

CHAPTER 16

BREATHWORK, RELAXATION AND YOGA

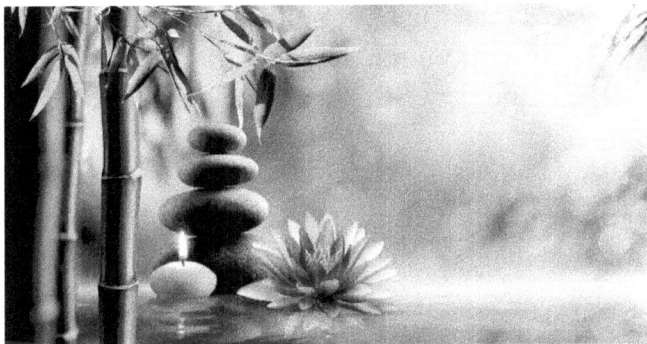

I love to travel. It is therapeutic for me to be free with myself and in nature. I went to Costa Rica for the first time one year before my mother passed away and took my father, two sons and my sister along.

We all really fell in love with Montezuma with its backward unpaved roads, raw old trees, colorful flowers, tropical fruits and animals including the curious monkeys. We all lapped up the ocean and sun and I felt as if this was like the "Garden of Eden." I go back yearly for yoga and breathwork retreats and to work privately on my own.

The instructor who did the breath work and yoga retreats really helped me breathe through other issues and come to peace with my family and close relationships. I cried at one of the sessions, grieving my mom's loss about six months after she passed away and it helped me so much with the grief process.

When I did the breathwork I felt tingling in my body and then I felt out of my body as more of an energetic entity and one with the universe. My friends and my sister all connected with the instructor as well and all of us had so much reverence for her as she helped all of us come to terms with some of our issues and to move forward in our lives.

Transformational Breathing involves retraining the body to breathe naturally like a child. Starting from the abdomen, the entire respiratory system is used in a relaxed and fully connected cycle.

By breathing this way, a natural self-healing response is triggered at three basic levels: physical body, mental/emotional field and spirit being. The technique works by combining body awareness, focused intent, affirmations, diagnostics and body mapping to create a well- balanced process that is perfectly suited to a 21st-century lifestyle.

The process is entirely natural and does not rely upon superimposing 'yet another breathing technique' upon already restricted patterns. Instead, its objective is to free up the body's mental and emotional fields such that the correct individual breathing pattern arises automatically from within. In this respect it re-trains us to employ what we already know; therein lies its simplicity, beauty, and greatest strength.

A breathing session is undertaken lying on the back and lasts for one hour. The first three to five sessions are carried out with the assistance of a trained facilitator. It is during this period that the majority of deep trauma is cleared from the subconscious.

Unlike most other breathing techniques, which are employed on an intermittent basis, this process of open, connected breathing is applicable on a continuous twenty-four hour a day basis. It is a process for life!

The human body is designed to take in 75% of its energy requirement through breathing; oxygen is the most fundamental unit of fuel that we take into our body. Further, we also eliminate 70% of our toxins via the breath; oxygen also cleanses the cells by oxidation and enables waste products to be carried back to the lungs via the bloodstream.

Given these basic facts, it is easy to see why learning to breathe correctly is one of the most fundamental things we can do to support and maintain our health and wellbeing.

Since we are not educated to become conscious of this fundamental metabolic process, over 90% of us are using less than 50% of our breathing capacity. The results of poor breathing practices and under-oxygenation are low energy levels, toxicity build-up, high stress and stagnant emotional states.

It is well accepted that long-term emotional stagnation eventually leads to physical and emotional disorders. Becoming a "conscious breather" can help our lives by fully oxygenating our system and maintaining a lucid state of emotional freedom.

Here's simple technique to experience relaxed abdominal breathing:

Sit back and put your hand on your belly, inhale and feel your abdomen rise; let your breath flow up to your chest, then, as you quickly exhale with a relaxed sigh, feel the chest and the abdomen fall; repeat this cycle 5 times without any pauses.

Note how you feel: more energized, lighter? Was it easy or difficult to access your abdominal muscles? Where are you tight and where are you relaxed? Could your breathing benefit from retraining?

All traditional cultures have recognized the value of conscious breathing practices, ranging from the pranayama practices of yoga to the Ha Breath of the Hawaiian Kahunas.

And there are a lot of breathing techniques to

choose from, including contemporary practices such as Holotropic Breath, Rebirthing, Clarity Breathwork, Vivation, Buteyko, Mézières etc.

It is very important to recognize that most ancient breathing practices, along with their modern counterparts, are either designed to induce altered states of consciousness, such as deep relaxation, bliss states, and out-of-body experiences, or they are intended to induce healing of a specific disorder, such as asthma, or birth and trauma release.

None of them are intended to teach us how to breathe correctly on a regular day-to-day basis. Transformational Breathing fills a very important gap in this respect.

Science tells us that at the heart of each cell we have a tiny atomic reactor that is constantly turning energy into matter (form building) and also releasing matter back into energy (conservation of energy).

While the mechanics of this process are well understood, the subtle mechanism that carries life energy to our cells has yet to be well described by science.

The key point to understand here is that the primary method that humans use to convert energy into form is through the BREATH. When we stop breathing we die; the more we breathe the more we live – it is that simple!

Correct Breathing

Having established the fundamental nature of the respiratory process in maintaining optimum energy levels, let us now look at how to breathe correctly for maximum benefit; that is to say starting in the abdomen and finishing in the upper chest.

Given that our strongest (primary) breathing muscles are the diaphragm, abdominal and intercostals, it makes good sense to use them as the prime movers in our breathing cycle.

During the first level of Transformational Breathing our body is re-trained to breathe starting from the abdomen; the seat of our personal power and subconscious. By inhaling in this way our abdomen is pushed outwards causing the diaphragm to extend downwards, opening up the lower part of our lungs.

This is extremely beneficial since it is the area with the highest density of alveoli – the small air sacs that transfer oxygen into our bloodstream.

Once it is full in the abdomen the breath wave moves across the diaphragm and up to the chest. It is within the diaphragm area that most restrictions are found. Known as the fear belt, it is the part of our body that carries most of our emotional traumas and muscular tension from fight or flight responses.

Once across the diaphragm, the breath wave travels up the chest and across the heart. The heart is the second area that is often congested, mostly with the tight muscular responses from repressed emotions such as loss, grief, hate, bitterness, love and ecstasy.

Once past the heart, the breath wave peaks into the upper chest/throat; the area of higher will. It is at the top of the breath wave that the secondary breathing muscles (scalenus, sternocleidomastoid, trapezius and pectoralis minor) come into play.

The secondary muscles provide balance and stability to our breathing system, but, being much lighter than the primaries, they also tire much more easily.

It is important to understand that the role of the primary and secondary breathing muscles should never be reversed. If they are (which is quite common), the result is tension, fatigue, neck, throat, jaw and upper back problems, breathlessness and an overall tendency to gasp on the out-breath – a factor which can lead to hyperventilation, in a desperate attempt to get more air.

By completely relaxing on the exhale, the natural elasticity of our ribs and muscular system is allowed to collapse our diaphragm and lungs, thus effortlessly expelling the air from our bodies.

No pauses are allowed between the out-/in-breath, for each pause represents holding on to the fear of letting go of negativity. Neither are there any pauses between the in-/out-breath since this represents a reluctance to engage fully with life. In practice, most of us have severe muscular restrictions to connected, open breathing and need quite a bit of encouragement to re-learn the basic mechanics.

It is at the level of our subconscious fears, doubts and insecurities that much of our resistance to breathing lies. By using a hands-on approach, a lot of these deeply embedded issues can be easily changed.

For example, by pressing on the fear release point (the muscle located just below the sternal notch) a lot of old issues can be quickly integrated, without having to know the intellectual content of the issues involved.

The second level of Transformational Breathing works on mind and feeling; in this case, the breath works as a connective link between our conscious and subconscious mind.

By using a focused intention, such as 'I connect to my personal power', or 'I connect to my life purpose, abundance, health, etc.', the mental and emotional blockages that prevent the manifestation of such an intent start to clear.

This process of integration works by a mechanism known as Entrainment; when high-frequency energy is brought into the body via the breath, the lower frequency mental/emotional (energetic) issues become excited to vibrate at a higher rate and thus are released more easily.

In order to understand this very important level more deeply it is necessary to have a clear picture of the relationship between breathing, energy, feeling, and emotion.

As we breathe, our life force or energy (called Prana or Chi by the Eastern philosophies) is drawn into our body. Interwoven upon this life force are our feelings, which arise in response to life experiences. The free-flowing movement of these feelings within our being is called emotion, energy motion or e-motion for short.

When we restrict the expression of our e-motions, by drawing away from intense feelings and limiting our self-expression, we create stuck energy states, which, since they have no place to go, convert into more dense states, typically re-appearing as the neuroses and physical illnesses of our modern world.

These disorders are nothing more than stuck e-motions that have been converted into matter through our conscious and unconscious attempts to protect ourselves from the intensity of our feelings; in their place, we have created intense states of dis-ease and dis-order.

One way that we fend off these old feelings is to shut down our breathing mechanism. Re-teaching our bodies to breathe correctly can clear this self-limiting dynamic.

Spirit – Creating a Clear Pathway through Breath Work

As we clear our subconscious minds of self-limiting destructive beliefs, outmoded behavior patterns and repressed feelings and memories, our awareness automatically connects to our innate indwelling spirit. Transformational Breathing is a powerful integrator at this level.

As conscious breathers we connect more deeply to our intuition and inner guidance, our body reverts to a natural state of bliss and wellbeing; our consciousness is transformed, and we move effortlessly from a consciousness based on fear to one based on miracles.

During this phase, many practitioners report experiencing higher states of awareness, whilst at the same time staying well-grounded in their bodies.

Benefits – What's in it for Me?

Benefits accrue at all three levels of body, mind, and spirit simultaneously and often at a level beyond conscious awareness.

While no specific medical claims are made, nearly all known disorders have been seen to respond favorably to conscious breathing, ranging from cancer to digestive disorders, migraines, heart and circulation problems, addictions, high blood pressure, sluggish immune system, depression, chronic fatigue, lack of self-empowerment, relationship problems, aggression and stress-related issues; the list is endless.

The simple truth is that complete oxygenation of our cellular system is essential for good health.

When oxygen levels increase in the blood the potential for dis-ease is reduced. High levels of oxygen kill germs, parasites, fungi, bacteria and viruses.

Nobel Prize Laureate Dr. Otto Warburg has proven that cancer cells live by fermentation. They are anaerobic and thus can only proliferate when cells are getting little or no oxygen. Their degenerative nature influences the cells around them as well. Dr. Warburg stated that if you deprive a cell of 60% of its oxygen it will turn cancerous.

This discovery has been instrumental in recent treatments for cancer and other incurables. Placed alongside the empirical observation that over 50% of us breathe at less than 30% capacity, it is not surprising that there are such a large number of cancer cases in society.

Oxygen is also essential for the biological release of such secretions as endorphins, serotonin, neu-

DR. BARBARA GORDON-COHEN, D.O.

ropeptides and hormones. These organic chemicals produce blissful and euphoric states and are normally released during peak experiences such as intense athletic activity, appreciation of a beautiful landscape, making love, a massage or a tender embrace.

These natural secretions are more powerful and far healthier than any artificial substance that is taken to get high.

Correct breathing is also a significant self-help tool for those applying oxygen healing therapies to such issues as immune disorders, cardiovascular diseases, cancer, HIV/AIDS, candida, and others.

Even childbirth can be transformed from a trauma into an ecstatic event by breathing with the contractions and not against them.

Equally so, asthma sufferers can enjoy a better life by learning that it is safe to let go of the exhale and that there is another breath coming on the in-breath. They learn that it is safe to breathe!

When I was first feeling anxiety, I knew that I needed to get help as the physical discomfort of chest pain, palpitations, feeling weak and shaky were overwhelming.

I felt raw and fragile and thus began cognitive behavioral therapy combined with psycho-analysis which enabled me to become a conscious human being. I began the process of understanding why I was so driven in my life and why I overextended myself when it came to care for others.

I learned to let go and am still always conscious of this process as I used to always feel as though I wanted control.

I think we all want control, but we really do not have any control. My lesson was to work to my potential, learn to take care of myself and to not be attached to any outcome as the outcome is beyond anyone's control. I learned to be in the moment as much as I could be and to take the time to breathe, meditate and enjoy everything as if it's my last day.

This concept is easy to say and hard to carry out, but it is my conscious decision to implement this way of thinking into my life and bring it into action.

I learned to let go of doing certain chores and then they were eventually done by others in my family or if they were not done I would let it be.

The more I let go the more liberated I became, and the tension started to dissipate.

Control issues are old patterns that can recur. Awareness of these patterns allows me to monitor my thought process and respond with positive affirmations to change the old patterns of behavior.

I have to say getting older, in general, makes us conscious and wiser. There is a certain inner peace as one becomes conscious and it's such an amazing feeling.

Cognitive Behavioral Therapy

Another powerful way to access the subconscious mind can be found through Cognitive Behavioral Therapy or CBT, which is a form of psychotherapy originally designed to treat depression but is now used to treat a number of mental disorders.

It works to solve current problems and change unhelpful thinking and behavior through therapy based on a combination of basic behavioral and cognitive principles. Most therapists often treat patients dealing with anxiety and depression through a blend of cognitive and behavioral therapy.

This technique acknowledges that there may be behaviors that cannot be controlled through rational thought but are instead based on prior conditioning from the environment and other external and/or internal stimuli.

It is different from the more traditional, psycho-analytical approach, where therapists look for the unconscious meaning behind the behaviors and then diagnose the patient.

CBT can be effective for a variety of conditions,

including mood, anxiety, personality disorders, eating disorders, addiction, dependence, tics, and psychotic disorders. CBT has also been shown to be worthwhile in treating chronic low back pain and fibromyalgia.

CHAPTER 17

NUTRITION

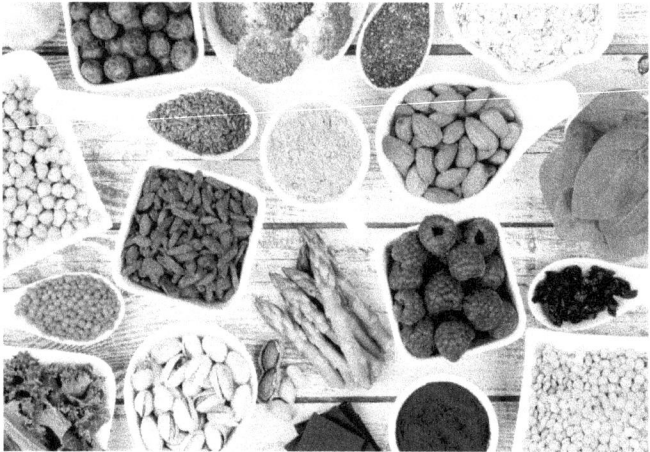

We've all heard of the phrase, "we are what we eat". Today this is even more so prevalent as we are living in a toxic environment. We have to deal with the elements of electromagnetic fields, pollution, pesticides, antibiotics and hormones injected into animals.

It's no wonder why there is so much cancer in the world and yet conventional medicine still does not address these issues.

What's Up with Gluten?

I have many patients who are sensitive to gluten (wheat, rye, barley, spelt) that come to my office with various complaints such as muscle pain, psoriasis, abdominal cramps, bloating, diarrhea, fatigue, eczema, depression, brain fog, itching skin, anxiety, hyperactivity, and under-active thyroid.

The combination of stress and the inflammatory properties of gluten can cause this intolerance.

Gluten and Inflammation

Did you know that there are other ingredients in wheat that are worth avoiding? Wheat is bad news for reasons that have nothing to do with gluten.

The Basics

Wheat is a grain with calories that come mostly from carbohydrates, but wheat also contains a few problem proteins such as wheat germ agglutinin and amylase trypsin inhibitor that create issues for a good percentage of those who ingest wheat.

What's wrong with wheat?

Wheat problems aren't restricted to people with Celiac disease.

The most important problem with wheat is celiac disease, an autoimmune reaction provoked by gluten and treatable with a gluten-free diet. 30-40% of people have the genetic background to potentially develop celiac disease, but only about 1-3% of people actually do – it's not clear why but it may have something to do with gut bacteria imbalance.

Most people know that celiac disease requires absolutely strict avoidance of all gluten. But a lot of people also think that if you don't have celiac disease, you're completely in the clear. This is not true.

There has been a recent increased interest in non-celiac gluten sensitivity (NCGS). Plenty of people have documented sensitivities to gluten that aren't actually celiac disease (but instead a different immune reaction involved).

There's also the overlapping problem of other proteins in wheat – wheat germ agglutinin and amylase trypsin inhibitors which are not the same thing as gluten and you can be sensitive to them regardless of how your body handles gluten.

Gut Inflammation

Inflammation is the natural response of your immune system to injury. The proteins in wheat are gut irritants and can cause an inflammatory response.

The most common case is the inflammation

caused by gluten in people with celiac disease or non-celiac gluten sensitivity is related to protein in gluten products.

Amylase trypsin inhibitors (ATIs for short) can provoke an inflammatory immune response in the GI tract by stimulating immune cells. This occurs in people regardless of whether they have celiac disease or not.

Increased Intestinal Permeability

Inflammation in the gut contributes to a problem called intestinal permeability also known as "leaky gut syndrome". The gut has a very complex system of "border control" that lets digested food into your bloodstream (this is how you get nutrients from it) while keeping everything else out.

Every day, you swallow millions of random viruses, bacteria, indigestible molecules like dust, and other stuff that needs to go out the other end, not into your bloodstream. Inflammation in the gut messes up that system of border control. It loosens the junctions between cells in the gut wall so too much stuff can pass through.

On top of inflammation leading to increased permeability, gluten accelerates this process by stimulating the release of a protein called zonulin.

Zonulin independently contributes to loosening the junctions between cells in the gut. Add together the inflammation and the zonulin, and wheat has a powerful effect on gut permeability, which is really a problem. Intestinal permeability is an essential factor in the development of auto-immune diseases.

Double Trouble: Wheat Germ Agglutinin

Another one for the non-Celiac crowd: wheat germ agglutinin is an inflammatory, immune-disrupting protein found in wheat and despite the similar name it isn't the same thing as gluten.

Wheat germ agglutinin can provoke an inflamma-tory response in gut cells and disturb the natural immune barrier in the gut, making the gut more permeable to things that don't belong in your blood. All kinds of stuff can get into the blood-stream even though it shouldn't be there.

Included in that stuff is... gluten!

Specifically, gliadin, which is a component of gluten. Once it's inside your bloodstream, gliadin runs into your immune system, and that's where the problems really start, in the form of molecular mimicry.

Molecular mimicry works like this: some foreign thing gets into the bloodstream. The immune system forms antibodies against it.

So far, so good: that's how the immune system is supposed to work.

But if that foreign thing looks enough like your own body's tissue, then the antibodies formed to fight it might start attacking your own body as well.

Gluten-related inflammation may also be a factor in the development of Crohn's Disease, another autoimmune gut disease. In a study of patients with inflammatory bowel disease (Crohn's Disease and ulcerative colitis), a gluten-free diet helped many people who tried it.

Increased Vulnerability to non-Celiac Autoimmune Diseases

If you go digging into the research on celiac disease and gluten, you'll find a bunch of studies linking it to all kinds of other autoimmune diseases, including autoimmune thyroid disorders, type 1 diabetes, fibro-myalgia (for both celiac disease and non-celiac gluten sensitivity!), rheumatoid arthritis, autoimmune liver disease, and a couple different autoimmune skin diseases.

The common factor here might be the gluten.

Wheat gluten is a major potential trigger of Type 1 Diabetes (that's the autoimmune type, not the diet-and-lifestyle type). Obesity and Type 2 Diabetes also have autoimmune components.

Damage to the Gut Flora

The gut flora, is the collection of friendly bacteria that live in your gut and help to regulate your immune system, control intestinal permeability, digest your food, synthesize nutrients like vitamin K2 (That help absorb calcium into the bones) send hunger/fullness signals to your brain, and prevent infections.

Gastrointestinal Symptoms

For people who do not have celiac disease, gluten may still cause immediate and severe symptoms (diarrhea and/or constipation, heartburn, pain, bloating, gas, stools that smell awful and sometimes vomiting.

Brain Symptoms

Brain fog and fatigue are symptoms of both celiac disease and non-celiac gluten sensitivity.

On a more serious note, the gut inflammation and microbiome disturbances involved in the immune-inflammatory response to gluten may increase vulnerability to dementia and Alzheimer's disease.

Autoimmunity in general (whether it's celiac disease or some other gluten-related autoimmunity) may be involved in depression.

This doesn't mean that gluten is the cause of all mental health problems or that eliminating gluten will cure them. Mental health is complicated and there are all kinds of factors to consider. The point is that in some people, gluten may be one of them.

Skin Symptoms

The most famous cause of gluten-related skin problems is celiac disease, which can cause a skin disease called dermatitis herpetiformis. Symptoms include an itchy, red rash with raised blisters that can be similar to eczema or psoriasis.

I personally did not have any gluten issues that I was aware of until after my mother passed away. Our family was under a lot of stress taking care of her and watching her fighting for her life with a diagnosis of leukemia. I started to get eczema on my forehead and over my eyebrows, but I did not recognize this as gluten sensitivity because I was so focused on my mother's health.

About 3 months after her death and subsequently three weeks later, my father having three strokes, I became aware that I had some sort of problem.

After the Jewish Holidays and all the Challah (braided bread) I ate, I started to get pressure in my bowels and cramping. I felt the sensation of wanting to have a bowel movement as well as pressure in my low back. My eczema was in my scalp and over my eyebrows.

I thought to myself maybe I am sensitive to wheat as I did have a lot of wheat products over the holidays. Lab tests showed that my gliadin anti-bodies (a test for gluten sensitivity and celiac) were positive.

I stopped all gluten and within two weeks all my symptoms cleared. I no longer had eczema or digestive issues. If I do cheat and have a little glu-ten I will usually have some nausea the next morning and some eczema. I try very hard to stay away from gluten as the digestive symptoms are intolerable.

I have had some quite amazing stories from my patients about symptoms that were related to gluten.

I had one patient who came in com-plaining of her skin itching so severely she was in agony. She had gone to the dermatologist and they did a biopsy, and all came back normal.

The doctor gave her cortisone with-out relief and then she developed joint pain in every joint that she could not move. She then went to the rheumatologist who did a battery of lab tests including gluten antibodies and everything came back negative.

She came back to my office and I told her even if the gluten test is normal you can still be sensitive to gluten. I told her to go off gluten for four weeks. She was also scheduled for surgery for a partial tear of her rotator cuff in her shoulder.

She reported back to me that in two weeks all her symptoms were gone including her shoulder pain, so she cancelled her surgery. We were both impressed.

I had another patient who had pain in between her shoulder blades and I had treated her osteopathically but the muscle pain was still there. I told her to go off wheat and her symptoms completely resolved.

Another patient was complaining of a chronic sore throat. He had been to the ears, nose and throat (ENT) doctor and had his throat checked by a scope and there were no findings except redness in the throat.

His throat cultures and labs were normal.

I did applied kinesiology and he was found to have a weakness to gluten so I told him to stop all gluten. He reported back to me that all his symptoms disappeared.

Recently I had a patient who had severe oozing and bleeding psoria-sis. His diet was horrible. I did applied kinesiology and he tested weak for sugar, gluten, citrus, and soy. He stopped these foods and one week later his psoriasis was 90% better.

So many people are intolerant to gluten that the supermarkets and health food stores are now carrying gluten free products.

It is important to note though that some of these gluten free products are not so healthy as they are high in potato starch, tapioca and sugar which is not good for blood sugar and weight loss.

You really have to read the labels and they should say no GMO.

GMO means a "genetically modified organism" altered by the techniques of genetic engineering so that its DNA contains one or more genes not normally found there.

Again, our body does not know what to do with unnatural food. Our cells and immune system do not know how to process these foods and we start producing antibodies to attack these foods causing similar reactions to the gluten intolerance.

There is clearly something going on with wheat that is not well known by the general public.

It goes far and beyond organic versus nonorganic, gluten or hybridization because even conventional wheat triggers no symptoms for some who eat wheat in other parts of the world.

Wheat Plant Toxicity

For quite some time, I secretly harbored the notion that wheat in the United States must, in fact, be genetically modified. GMO wheat secretly invading the North American food supply seemed the only thing that made sense and could account for the varied experiences I was hearing about.

I reasoned that it couldn't be the gluten or wheat hybridization. Gluten and wheat hybrids have been consumed for thousands of years. It just didn't make sense that this could be the reason for so many people suddenly having problems with wheat and gluten in general in the past 5-10 years.

The bad news is that the problem lies with the

way wheat is grown and harvested by conventional wheat farmers.

Common wheat harvest protocol in the US is to drench the wheat fields with the herbicide **Roundup**® several days before the combine harvesters work through the fields as the practice allows for an earlier, easier and bigger harvest.

Pre-harvest application of the Roundup® or other herbicides containing the deadly active ingredient glyphosate to wheat and barley as a desiccant was suggested as early as 1980. It has since become routine over the past 15 years and is used as a drying agent 7-10 day before harvest within the conventional farming community.

Monsanto, the manufacturer of Roundup® claims that application to plants at over 30% kernel moisture result in Roundup® uptake by the plant into the kernels. Farmers like this practice because Roundup® kills the wheat plant allowing an earlier harvest.

Using Roundup® on wheat crops throughout the entire growing season and even as a desiccant just prior to harvest may save the farmer money and increase profits, but it is devastating to the health of the consumer who ultimately consumes the glyphosate residue laden wheat kernels.

The currently accepted view is that glyphosate is not harmful to humans or any mammals. However, just because Roundup® doesn't kill you immediately doesn't make it nontoxic. In fact, the active ingredient in Roundup® lethally disrupts the all-important shikimate pathway found in beneficial gut microbes which is responsible for synthesis of the critical amino acids – phenylalanine, tyrosine, and tryptophan.

Friendly gut bacteria, also called probiotics, play a critical role in human health. Gut bacteria aid digestion, prevent permeability of the gastrointestinal tract (which discourages the development of autoimmune disease), synthesize vitamins and provide the foundation for robust immunity.

In essence:

Roundup® significantly disrupts the functioning of beneficial bacteria in the gut and contributes to permeability of the intestinal wall and consequent expression of autoimmune disease symptoms.

As a result, humans exposed to glyphosate through use of Roundup® in their community or through ingestion of its residues on industrialized food products become even more vulnerable to the damaging effects of other chemicals and environmental toxins they encounter!

What's worse is that the negative impact of glyphosate exposure is slow and insidious over months and years as inflammation gradually gains a foothold in the cellular systems of the body.

The consequences of this systemic inflammation are most of the diseases and conditions associated with the Western lifestyle:

- Gastrointestinal disorders
- Obesity
- Diabetes
- Heart Disease
- Depression
- Autism
- Infertility
- Cancer
- Multiple Sclerosis
- Alzheimer's disease

And the list goes on and on and on.

The bottom line is that avoidance of conventional wheat in the US is absolutely imperative even if you don't currently have a gluten allergy or wheat sensitivity.

The increase in the amount of glyphosate applied to wheat closely correlates with the rise of celiac disease and gluten intolerance. The effects of deadly glyphosate on your biology are so insidious that lack of symptoms today means literally nothing.

What's Up with Dairy?

I personally had a dairy allergy as a baby and my mother told me I would have a skin rash if given dairy. What I could remember about dairy was that I craved it. I loved cheese, quiches, pizza, spaghetti with cheese, Italian dishes with ricotta cheese and parmesan.... oh, so good.

I had terrible allergies as a child. I was allergic to cats, mold, dust and mites and ragweed during the fall season. I would have a stuffy nose, sneezing, itching nose, throat and eyes. The more stress I was under the worse my allergies got.

When I moved away from my home which, was a 10-minute drive to the beach my allergies did improve. I was no longer near mold or the cat. I still had a stuffy nose and my friends would say that I had a nasal voice. I continued to eat dairy and the stuffy nose continued as well.

When I learned that dairy can cause nasal congestion, earaches, coughing, gas, bloating, diarrhea, and fatigue, I decided to halt my diary intake. I noticed that I was no longer stuffy or fatigued.

I can still have dairy occasionally without any side effects, but I use coconut milk and almond milk instead of cow's milk. Sometimes I treat myself to goat's milk and cheese which is less allergenic and is also not massed produced using hormones.

Did you know that...

Milk is the foundation of heart disease and the explanation for America's number one killer.

Eighty-nine percent of America's dairy cows have the leukemia virus.

Milk is the reason that one out of six American women will develop cancer of the breast. A recent study shows women exposed to bovine leukemia virus, a routine presence in bulk milk tanks at large dairy farms, are 3.1 times more likely to develop breast cancer than women whose tissue was not subject to the virus.

Milk is a factor in the data showing that twenty-five million American women over the age of forty have been diagnosed with bone crippling arthritis and osteoporosis. These females have been drinking more than two to 4 cups of milk per day for their entire adult lives.

Calcium in milk is not adequately absorbed and milk consumption is the probable cause of osteoporosis.

Simply put osteoporosis results from calcium loss, not insufficient calcium intake. And dairy products, because of their high protein content, promote calcium loss. Studies examining the incidence of osteoporosis have found that high consumption of dairy products is associated with high rates of osteoporosis. If you want strong bones, don't drink milk.

Milk is responsible for allergies, colic, colitis, earaches, colds and congestion in young children.

Research indicates that a bovine protein in milk destroys the insulin-producing beta cells of the pancreas, causing diabetes. And milk allergies are very common in children and cause sinus problems, diarrhea, constipation, fatigue and they are a leading cause of the chronic ear infections that plague up to 40% of all children under the age of six.

Milk allergies are also linked to iron-deficiency anemia in infants, childhood behavioral problems and to the disturbing rise in childhood asthma.

The Food and Drug Administration (FDA) used to allow a small amount of antibiotics in milk until scientists recognized that consumers should not be drinking a fluid containing antibiotics. In 1990, the one part per hundred- million antibiotic residue in milk standard was increased by one-hundred times to one part per million.

As a result, new strains of bacteria developed, immune to the 52 different antibiotics found in milk.

Antibiotics are less effective because Americans have been drinking milk and eating dairy products containing increased amounts of these powerful drugs and, in addition, new strains of emerging diseases.

Milk Alternatives

COCONUT MILK

Compared to cow's milk, coconut milk is simple to make, easy to digest and contains an abundance of nutrients:

Coconut milk is high in magnesium that helps to keep your blood pressure at a normal level. The combination of calcium and magnesium in coconut milk also keeps muscle and nerves from becoming overstimulated.

Coconut milk helps fight viruses and infection due to its lauric acid content that is converted to monolaurin in your body. This compound contains antiviral and antibacterial properties.

The manganese in coconut milk helps you me-tabolize glucose in the body to help the metabolism working at the optimum level. Manganese can also help to prevent osteoporosis, PMS, inflammation and vitamin absorption.

Coconut milk is high in saturated fat, but this type of fat raises the HDL or good cholesterol while dairy based products raise the LDL or bad cholesterol. The fat in coconut milk is easy for your body to metabolize which will lower your cholesterol levels overall.

The selenium in coconut milk acts as an antioxidant that will help to reduce free radicals that can cause joint inflammation, heart disease and cancer.

You can consume coconut milk or apply it directly to the skin to create a smoother texture because the fat in this product will help your skin lock in moisture. After cleansing your skin, place a layer of coconut milk on your skin for 15 minutes then rinse it away for best results.

Placing a layer of coconut milk on sunburned skin will help to moisturize this area and soothe the pain.

Massage coconut oil into the scalp and gently down the hair strands then wrap your hair in a towel and leave the oil in place for a couple hours. This will allow the coconut oil to deeply penetrate your hair and moisturize it to give your hair a deep conditioning treatment.

Other Benefits of Coconut Milk:

As a substitute for cream in coffee, coconut milk contains high electrolytes, sodium, potassium and chloride that will help keep you hydrated. This is much healthier than consuming high amounts of dairy products each day.

Those that are lactose intolerant or practice a vegan diet often use coconut milk in place of dairy products in baked goods. Coconut milk is thicker than many other milk substitutes to help maintain the desired consistency of your dessert, so vegan desserts do not lack the bulk that the original recipe would have.

ALMOND MILK

Another great dairy-free milk substitute is almond milk even though it's important to note that it doesn't provide as much protein or calcium to be a complete substitute, so make sure you receive adequate amounts from other sources. One cup only has one gram of protein.

Almond milk helps with weight management. One cup of almond milk contains only 60 calories, as opposed to 146 calories in whole milk. It makes for a great substitute that will help you lose or maintain your current weight.

There's no cholesterol or saturated fat in almond milk. It's also low in sodium and high in healthy fats (such as omega fatty acids, typically found in fish), which helps to prevent high blood pressure and heart disease.

Almond milk offers 25 percent of the recommended amount of vitamin D, reducing your risk for arthritis and osteoporosis and improving your immune function.

Almond milk contains 50 percent of the recommended daily amount of vitamin E, which contains antioxidant properties essential to your skin's health, such as protecting it against sun damage.

Almond milk (with no additives) is low in carbs, which means it won't significantly increase your blood sugar levels, reducing your risk for diabetes. Because of its low glycemic index, your body will use the carbs as energy, so the sugars aren't stored as fat.

Although almond milk only contains 1 gram of protein per serving it contains plenty of B vitamins important for muscle growth and healing.

Almond milk contains almost one gram of fiber per serving, which is important for healthy digestion.

Lactose intolerance impacts about 25% of the US population, which means they have difficulty digesting the sugar in cow's milk. This makes almond milk a suitable, lactose-free substitute.

Almond milk doesn't taste like cow's milk, perfect for those who are turned off by the taste. It has its own unique flavor many describe as being light and crisp. Bonus: it's versatile, meaning you can use it instead of cow's milk in recipes that require it. While it won't have the same taste, it will have the same consistency.

Knowing that you don't have to refrigerate almond milk means you'll be more likely to take it with you to work, or on a camping trip.

It's perfectly fine at room temperature which makes it a convenient, nutritious staple to pack, automatically upping your daily intake of all the fabulous nutrients.

CHAPTER 18

SUGAR

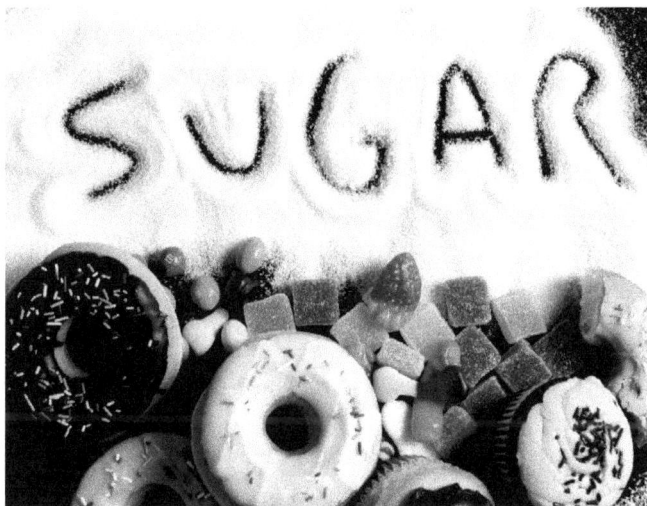

Why is there such a bad rap on sugar?

There is an epidemic of diabetes, cardio-vascular disease, cancer and obesity in the world. Not only that, but of my patients who have constantly been on antibiotics, steroids or under a lot of stress, eating sugar seems to make them weaker and exhausted.

Too much sugar makes the pancreas work harder. Insulin production is then increased and after a while, the receptor sites that bind to insulin get exhausted and become less efficient so the sugar increases in the blood stream increasing the incidence of diabetes.

Diabetes is a silent killer which increases vascular disease, nerve disease, loss of vision, and kidney disease.

If one is under stress cortisol is increased by the adrenal glands which stimulate sugar to increase in the bloodstream. Then the pancreas has to work harder to produce insulin to draw the sugar into the liver.

One can end up with hypoglycemia or low blood sugar and a sensation of starvation can occur when eating too much sugar and under stress.

Then weight starts to increase around the belly and you end up with metabolic syndrome. Metabolic syndrome increases belly fat, triglycerides, cholesterol and can eventually cause diabetes.

Vascular disease as a result of diabetes increases the risks of heart attack, stroke, visual loss, amputations, leg cramping, and pain.

Many of us are passive consumers in our society. We tend not to look at food product labels to see the amount of sugar in what we eat. Anything over 12 grams of sugar is just too high and will put you at risk down the road.

There are many who crave sugar and are "sugar" addicts. They like the "up" feeling of sugar but eventually crash. I find many of my patients who crave sugar go through withdrawal when going off sugar. They may experience fatigue, moodiness, diarrhea, shaky feeling, and inability to concentrate until the sugar withdrawal ends. This may take up to a week.

I find that many who are sugar addicts have a history of family alcohol addiction and even if they are not alcoholics, their parents or grandparents are often alcoholics. They have the gene that craves the sugar that is also in alcohol, so these people may not be alcoholics but rather sugar addicts.

I had one patient who was very obese complaining of fatigue and moodiness. She admitted she was a sugar addict and had a history in her family of her grandfather being an alcoholic. When I told her, she had to go off sugar, she cried. But she was determined and after withdrawal for one week, she felt great. Her energy improved and the moodiness completely disappeared.

I have other patients who have been on antibiotics or steroids consistently, end up with yeast infections or bowel problems. The yeast overgrowth from the medication absolutely love sugar and feed off of it and grow in your body.

Then one can have symptoms of fatigue, brain fog, diarrhea, intestinal gas and bloated feeling, headaches, and frequent yeast infections. They have to get off sugar, so the yeast starts to miss the sugar, get a Herxheimer reaction where they feel sicker than ever for about one to three weeks and then they start feeling better.

Probiotics, digestive enzymes, and glutamine are then introduced to help strengthen the gut flora and improve a "leaky bowel" from destruction due to medications and yeast overgrowth. This healing takes time and a lot of patience.

Sometimes anti-yeast medication is necessary to destroy the excess yeast that is feeding on sugar, fermented food, mold, and carbohydrates.

The diet then must be cleaned up and even sugary fruits have to be avoided in this situation.

They need to go on a yeast free diet which means no sugar, no moldy fruits and vegetables, no yeast, no alcohol, no bread, or hard cheeses. This is not a forever situation, but it could take up to one year to really heal the gut.

I personally had severe problems with sugar in my first year of medical school. When I ate sugar like ice cream which was a favorite of mine, I had to go to sleep within one hour.

I also remember after having my fourth child that when I ate a bagel I would get fatigued as well and would have to lie down. Now I can have sugar in moderation as my stress is not as high and also because I meditate, and my life has become more balanced with exercise and rest.

I try to avoid as much sugar as I can as I know a sugar-free diet may prevent cancer and vascular diseases. I prefer to eat fruit over any other sweet food. The healthier you eat the more you want to eat this way and the desire to eat sweets diminishes.

Cancer feeds on sugar which increases cancer growth and metastases. I believe we can live in harmony with cancer cells if our diet and our lifestyles are balanced.

I have a cancer patient who has been living for over ten years since being diagnosed, due to eating healthy, juicing, taking antioxidants and anti-tumor growth herbs, without chemotherapy, radiation, and surgery.

He could not afford any of the conventional treatments due to a lack of insurance. He did everything in his power to beat cancer and he is still alive and working.

I had a colleague who had the same cancer who had surgery, radiation, chemotherapy, and hormone treatment. He did not live beyond six years, suffered greatly and had no quality of life.

Avoiding sugar, meat and coffee and a diet composed of fresh fruit and vegetables will make the body more alkaline. A shift to an alkaline terrain will inhibit the spread of cancer cells.

My father was obese because he was a food addict. He developed diabetes and hypertension and needed medication. He insisted on eating the wrong foods and did not change his lifestyle.

He ended up suffering two strokes after my mother passed away because the stress of her death put him over the edge.

He was a walking time bomb and he did it to himself. He has lost 70 pounds since the strokes and as a result, does not need blood pressure meds, his diabetic meds have been reduced in half, and he does not snore anymore. Too bad he had to experience a stroke before applying the changes that were necessary.

My husband and I were walking one evening and

a man in his sixties was walking past us. He said he walked daily because he wanted to prove his doctors wrong. They told him he was a diabetic and he would have to go on medication for the rest of his life. He lost over fifty pounds and his sugar is now normal. He told us he would prove them wrong and he did it! You can do it too!

DR. BARBARA GORDON-COHEN, D.O.

CHAPTER 19

CAFFEINE

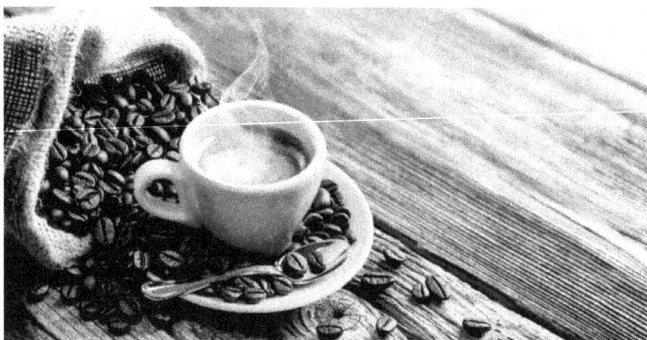

I personally feel that if one is under a lot of stress they should limit ingesting caffeine as the adrenal glands are producing a lot of cortisol, and norepinephrine, the "the flight and fight hormones".

The production of these hormones alone can cause palpitations and the caffeine in conjunction with the adrenals producing these hormones can also cause chest pain, irregular heartbeats, numbness, insomnia and ultimately, exhaustion.

Mayo Clinic research shows that consuming more than 500-600 mg (more than 2-4 cups of coffee) of caffeine a day may lead to insomnia, nervousness, restlessness, irritability, an upset stomach, a fast heartbeat, and even muscle tremors. However, previous research has linked even more moderate amounts of caffeine to negative health effects.

Another study has suggested that consuming 300 mg of caffeine a day during pregnancy may increase the risk of low birth weight babies, while other research suggests that drinking four cups of coffee a day may increase the risk of early death.

The effects of caffeine can vary in each individual, which may explain why there are mixed messages surrounding whether caffeine is good or bad for us. Some people may have difficulty sleeping or experience tremors or stress with relatively low caffeine intake i.e. as much as one cup a day.

If you suffer from anxiety disorder and insomnia, caffeine can make it worse.

Some people can become physically dependent on caffeine and withdrawal can trigger symptoms such as a headache, fatigue, drowsiness, depression, irritability, concentration difficulties, nausea, and vomiting.

In medical school I became dependent on 2 cups of coffee a day. Coffee increased my ability to concentrate and I experienced feelings of euphoria. Once the coffee wore off, I desired sleep, experienced heart palpitations and eventually numbness in my hands and feet.

The combination of stress and caffeine depleted my energy reserves.

Once I stopped ingesting coffee, I suffered with a 3-day headache and an inability to concentrate: a detoxification reaction. Once I completed the detoxification process, I was able to make it through my remaining tenure in medical school and residency.

Other than coffee, caffeine is commonly consumed through tea, soft drinks – particularly energy drinks – and chocolate. It is also found in some prescription and nonprescription drugs, such as cold, allergy and pain medication.

Caffeine's Potential Health Benefits

For the person who has Attention Deficit Disorder or ADHD, caffeine can help with focus and have a calming effect. And, like many other reinforcers, caffeine is associated with various subjective effects like increased well-being, sociability, and feelings of energy and alertness.

Some studies have suggested that drinking three or four cups of coffee a day may reduce the risk of liver, mouth and throat cancer.

One study suggests that consuming three cups of coffee a day may reduce the risk of liver cancer by 50%, while another study suggests that drinking four cups a day could cut the risks of mouth and throat cancer by 50%.

Caffeine consumption has also been associated with positive effects on the brain.

A Harvard study suggests that drinking between two and four cups of coffee a day may reduce suicide risk in adults, while more recent research found that ingesting 200 mg of caffeine each day may boost long-term memory.

Other studies have also suggested that caffeine intake may protect against type 2 diabetes,

Parkinson's disease, cardiovascular disease and stroke.

Wow what a mixed rap!

CHAPTER 20

ARTIFICIAL SWEETENERS

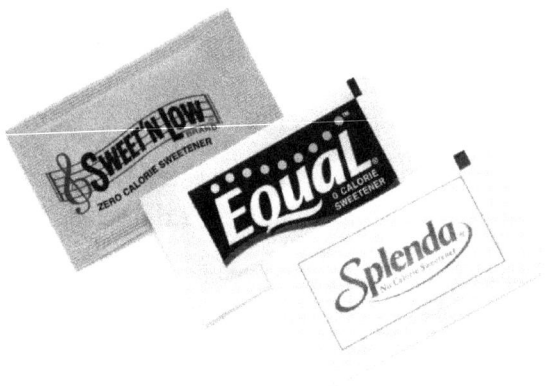

Have you been using artificial sweeteners in an effort to lose weight and cut calories? It's time to rethink that. Some of the worst ones to avoid are:

- Aspartame (Equal®, NutraSweet®, NatraTaste Blue®)

- Sucralose (Splenda®)

- Acesulfame K (ACE-K, Sunette®, Equal® Spoonful, Sweet One®, Sweet 'n Safe®)

- Saccharin (Sweet 'N Low®, Sweet Twin®), Xylitol, Sorbitol

Here's why:

1. Aspartame
(Equal®, NutraSweet®, NatraTaste Blue®)

The U.S. Food and Drug Administration approved aspartame nearly 35 years ago and it is currently used in more than 6,000 consumer foods and drinks, and over 500 prescription drugs and over-the-counter medications.

It hides in places we don't expect! Because aspartame isn't heat-stable, it's typically found in drinks and foods that haven't been heated.

A public health study recently concluded that aspartame has carcinogenic effects and that this artificial sweetener may also impair memory performance and increase oxidative stress in the brain.

In addition, if you are pregnant or nursing, avoid this dangerous artificial sweetener at all costs. Studies show women who consume artificial sweeteners during pregnancy or while breastfeeding can predispose babies to metabolic syndrome disorders, and obesity, later in life.

Common side effects of aspartame include headaches, migraines, mood disorders, dizziness and episodes of mania. Comprising phenylalanine, aspartic acid, and methanol, these substances can stay in the liver, kidneys, and brain for quite some time.

2. Sucralose (Splenda®)

Sucralose, derived from sugar, was originally introduced as a natural sugar substitute. But it is actually processed with chlorine, one of the most toxic chemicals on the planet!

Sucralose was originally found through the development of a new insecticide compound and wasn't originally intended to be consumed.

At 600 times sweeter than sugar, it's easy to see how the use of sucralose, or Splenda® (!), can contribute to an addiction for overly sweet foods and drinks.

3. Acesulfame K (ACE, ACE-K, Sunette®, Sweet One®, Sweet 'N Safe®)

Composed of a potassium salt that contains methylene chloride, Acesulfame K is routinely found in sugar-free chewing gum, alcoholic beverages, candies and even sweetened yogurts. It's often used in combination with aspartame and other non caloric sweeteners.

ACE K has undergone the least amount of scientific scrutiny even though long-term exposure to methylene chloride, the main chemical component, has been shown to cause nausea, mood problems, possibly some types of cancer, impaired liver and kidney function, problems with eyesight, and even autism.

It is heat-stable and routinely found in highly processed foods and baked goods. The human body can't break it down, and it's believed to negatively affect the metabolism.

4. Saccharin (Sweet 'N Low®)

In the 1970s, saccharin and other sulfa-based sweeteners were believed to possibly cause bladder cancer, and it was required to carry a warning label. Despite the FDA eventually removing the warning, many studies continue to link saccharin to serious health issues.

Sadly, it is the primary sweetener for children's medications, including chewable aspirin, cough syrup, and other over-the-counter and prescription medications. It's believed that saccharin contributes to photosensitivity, nausea, digestive upset, tachycardia and some types of cancer.

5. Xylitol (Erythritol, Maltitol, Mannitol, Sorbitol and other sugar alcohols that end in –itol)

Sugar alcohols aren't absorbed well by the body and can cause allergic reactions for those who have a sensitivity to it.

In addition, it has gastrointestinal side effects that include bloating, gas, cramping, and diarrhea. Its laxative effect is so pronounced that it's actually part of the chemical makeup for many over-the-counter laxatives.

Healthy Alternatives to Artificial Sweeteners

All-natural sweeteners – including maple syrup, coconut sugar, stevia, fruit purees, date syrup, Sucanat and raw honey – are great, healthy substitutions.

Keep packets of stevia with you so you don't have to resort to artificial sweeteners provided by restaurants and cafes.

Start working to retrain your palate to enjoy the natural sweetness of foods, not added sweeteners. Try adding other flavors like tangy, tart, warm and savory to please your palate. For example, vanilla, cocoa, licorice, nutmeg, and cinnamon enhance the flavor of foods, so you need less sweetness.

When you crave a sweet drink, sweeten your iced tea with honey, coconut sugar or even maple syrup for a twist. Replace foods with artificial sweeteners with fruit. Personally, I like to make chai tea, adding cinnamon, coconut milk and stevia which makes it such a nice treat.

America's obesity epidemic continues to grow and interestingly coincides with an increase in the widespread use of non-nutritive artificial sweeteners.

Research shows that artificial sweeteners don't really satiate you the way real foods do and instead leave you feeling less satisfied and more prone to eating and drinking more.

Some documented cases:

I have studied aspartame (NutraSweet®, Equal®) for more than 25 years because it caused a drastic personality change and intellectual deterioration in my daughter. She also developed epileptic-type seizures and began to lose the vision in both eyes. She consulted a neurologist, and he told her that she had temporal lobe epilepsy.

He began treating her with medication, but the medication didn't work, because the doctor was wrong in his diagnosis and he was treating her for a condition she didn't have! What she really had was a reaction to ASPARTAME.

To follow up, we took our daughter to Boston for special studies on her brain, and the doctors confirmed that it was NutraSweet® that had made her so sick.

They said that she had been totally misdiagnosed by a neurologist at the Clinical Research Center at the Massachusetts Institute of Technology and that she did not have temporal lobe epilepsy at all.

We also took her to a highly-respected ophthalmologist who explained why her vision loss was due to aspartame. She finally stopped drinking sodas containing aspartame, and had a complete recovery.

In the early 80s, I started having strange symptoms. Patchy numbness, ringing in ears, etc. I also was drinking Diet Coke®. In 1988 while at a staff meeting, my face went numb on the left side. It felt like netting coming across my face. Fortunately, I was in a hospital and was immediately taken to the emergency room.

To make a long story short, after years of people telling me I had MS, or other neurological symptoms, in

2008 I decided to listen to two of my co-workers – "Get off Diet Coke®". I did.

The medication I had to take is no longer needed, the burning sensation and the patch of numbness disappeared from all the other places. Now I do not touch anything with "light" on it.

Funny, I have not gained weight, so drinking Diet Coke was useless. I stick with the stevia drinks – I hope someday Coke will have to quit making that poison.

That is my story. Stay away from aspartame.

I have had terrible reactions to Splenda®. It feels like a heart attack – it's awful. Palpitations, tightness, shortness of breath, and it's, unfortunately, common. I really wish they'd do some better studies on this stuff. My personal opinion.

A Case History of Sucralose Poisoning

My close friend Melissa, a nutritionist and athletic trainer, shares her story of being "poisoned" by sucralose. She was among the hundreds of people each year who end up seriously ill because of artificial sweeteners. Here is her chilling account of her experience and what she had to endure to heal her body:

My throat had been swollen for a good three weeks by now – I had lost my voice and was waking up nightly with a cough and severe gut pain. I came home mid-morning from teaching a cycling class sat down on my couch and suddenly the room began to spin, and my body felt cemented to the couch. I had to struggle to call 911 – I thought I was having a stroke.

ER: IV drip of pain and anti-nausea meds – CAT scans, poked and scanned and scoped.

Diagnosis: Internal gut and vocal cord swelling – referred to GI doctor.

Mid-June: UCLA GI Dr and UCLA ENT – many tests, with contrast and without contrast, swallowed a camera – radio isotopes, etc. By this time, I had double vision and my eyeballs were shifting right to left uncontrollably along with a migraine that wouldn't let up and vertigo. I was housebound, crawling or sliding against the walls to move from place to place.

Diagnosis: GERD

By mid-July, I had been to the ER 5 times for uncontrollable pain. I was put on all kinds of antacids, and a battery of gut and migraine medicines. "Drink Ensure," the doctor said to me. Needless to say, I lost all faith in her and I stopped seeing her.

I was getting worse – all my symptoms were increasing as well as the pain. The pain was so bad that it was consuming me. I had a colonoscopy and an endoscopy (looking for stomach cancer, esophageal cancer).

The scopes revealed my gut lining was swollen and my small intestine inflamed with what looked like an abrasion.

Yet with all the meds, I was getting worse daily. I was now unable to move my bowels and needed more intervention. During all of this – I could only get liquids down and was drinking a meal replacement drink that I had started 8 months prior – thinking at least I'd get some protein and essential nutrients. I drank the drink three to four times a day. I couldn't digest anything, and the headache pain was unbearable.

I was finally referred to UCLA Neurology to the most brilliant doctor I had ever met. She thoroughly took my history and wanted to rewind to the past year. Her question was, "How can a perfectly healthy athletic woman, crash this badly?"

She asked me if I had done anything new and different in the past year. I told her about the weight loss supplements that I'd been consuming. I had bought a full package of protein drinks, bars, cereal and energy powders from a multi-level marketing company. I had been replacing two meals a day with the drink, eating the bars and using their cereal.

Unfortunately for me, I hadn't lost the body fat I was on a mission to lose on the program, but stayed on the drinks because I was feeling so sick that I couldn't hold down food. She asked me to bring her the products.

When I brought them to her – she looked at the ingredients – there was the answer – SUCRALOSE. She told me to stop using the products immediately. She told me that sucralose is a neurotoxin and that it crosses the blood-brain barrier. She told me that I was experiencing vestibular migraines in my gut and my head.

The only way I can describe what happened to my health is that I "face-planted." I went from being a super fit and active fitness profess-ional – cycling 60 miles a week, teaching 5 deep water aqua classes and full-time Pilates and personal training to being almost paralyzed.

I was unable to leave my house, unable to control the pain that took over my body, unable to walk or eat or sleep.

It was as if my life force was gone.

Debilitating gut and head pain, and vertigo had left me with no real medical diagnosis or answers and the inability to function in my life.

I spent 6 months on disability and watched my health continuously in a landslide. My spirit started to go too. Day in and day out, I sat on the porch doing everything I could to keep my brain active.

UCLA has what's known as East/West medicine. I was lucky enough to be referred there. I went through a series of acupuncture sessions and was told I had "Liver Yang Rising" and was put on a specific eating plan.

This plan included bitter cucumber and dandelion greens. I went a step further and did a lot of research. After all, I couldn't do anything but sit so I developed a plan of action for myself.

I threw out all the medicine and went on this green juice cleanse protocol:

Upon rising – A small glass of salt water – 4 oz. of pure organic aloe vera juice and a 30 billion CFU probiotic to heal my gut followed by an elixir of apple cider vinegar, goldenseal, oregano oil, turmeric, and pure organic apple juice mixed with water to alkalize and reduce inflammation, boost immunity and destroy yeast overgrowth, and unhealthy bacteria.

An hour later – Juices from organic greens, some sour fruits, and root veggies to alkalize my body and rebuild my immune system and deglyceri-nated licorice to heal my stomach lining.

An hour later – Organic plain Greek yogurt with acidophilus

2 hours later – cooked beets with dandelion greens and sips of bone broth to heal my gut and detox my liver. Magnesium, apple pectin, and vi-tamin C to relax my nervous system and increased killing off free radicals.

2 hours later – More juice with Moringa powder added and a few cooked egg whites on the side for protein and immune system boosting.

Ashwagandha capsules to strengthen adrenals.

DGL Licorice to soothe stomach and intestinal lining.

Dinner – Bone Broth and beets with dandelion to heal leaky gut and cleanse the liver.

Senna Tea to aid in regulating bowel movements.

Every evening – Coffee enema to cleanse the liver for about two weeks – then down to twice a week, then every other week – then once a month to every two months.

This was my routine for the next six months – adding what I could when I could. I was able to add in some boiled chicken and began to eat cooked greens and asparagus and learned that celery and cucumber were easily digested.

Medically, the next step was botox injections for my migraine pain – this was to be done every three months – 200 units or more, all over my head, neck and trapezius muscles. I continue on this treatment which has helped to ease the chronic pain pattern that my brain had established.

The DGL (deglycerinated licorice) was what weaned me off Prilosec. It's a great substitute and actually also helped heal my gut. I used baking soda and water as well if I had chest pain related to the gut.

Imagine – this was all brought on by sucralose. I learned that just 4 little yellow packets of sucralose can wipe out your intestinal flora.

The protein powder I was on also had maltodextrin which was washed with MSG. The supplement industry is unregulated, and consumers should only take those with third party clinical research.

I have taken my misfortune and am working in the field of nutrition and now in school to become a naturopath. I specialize in Leaky Gut Syndrome and Candida as well as weight loss and educating the masses on the ills of artificial sweeteners and processed foods. I had spoken with 5 different attorneys about suing the makers of Sucralose.

They said it would be like trying to take down the tobacco companies.

I found over 150 people in a chat room that had similar experiences to mine. One of them had tried to put together a class action suit and was getting threatening letters and a demand for cease and desist.

I hope that my story can serve to help others suffering from pain that is unexplained. I pray that I can reach as many families as possible and educate the head of the kitchen as to what healthy, fit eating is.

CHAPTER 21

THE HISTORY OF CRANIAL THERAPY

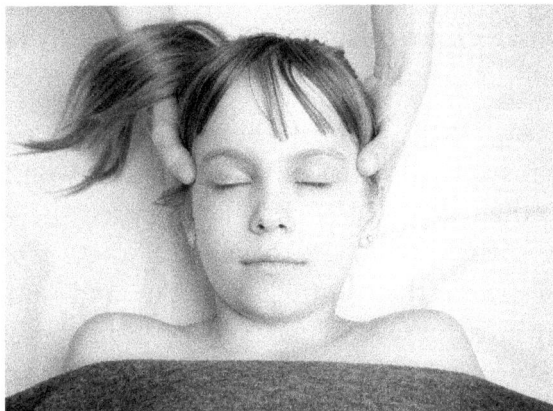

I have mentioned throughout this book cases where patients were totally cured with cranial treatments for newborns, children, and adults.

I have treated babies with acute and chronic ear infections, sinus infections, constipation, colicky babies, babies who have problems sucking or swallowing and babies who vomit or have reflux, neck issues (torticollis), structural problems, respiratory disorders, and digestive issues, with complete success.

I have helped adults with low back pain and sciatica, neck pain with radiating pain down the arm, TMJ, physical traumas and many other conditions.

The Founding Forefather of Cranial Therapy

William Garner Sutherland, D.O. (1873-1954) noticed when he was in Osteopathic Medical school a disarticulated skull in his anatomy lab. (a skull whose bones were separated).

He saw all the intricate bevels and grooves and sutures between the skull bones and he wondered why they were there. He asked himself the question – why did the creator make all these separate bones with their intricate shapes and sutures? Why was there not just one bone in the skull? How was the skull formed at birth and how did it develop?

He spent his whole life exploring the bones, the dura around the bones, and the cerebrospinal fluid within the spinal cord and brain and all the tissues of the body.

Dr. Sutherland did experiments to prove that the cranial mechanism exists. He studied the anatomy of the bones, dura, nerves, vessels, and spaces in the cranium (ventricles) that produce the cerebro-spinal fluid as well as the anatomy of the dura, (I call it saran wrap around the brain), that surround the brain and divide the brain into hemispheres upper and lower and right and left side.

He saw how the dura attaches firmly at the junction of the head and neck and upper neck and that loosely travels down the spine to attach firmly to the second segment of the sacrum (or end of the spine)

He studied:

1. the fluctuation of the Cerebral spinal fluid

2. the inherent motility of the CNS

3. the mobility between the cranial and spinal dural membranes

4. the articular mobility of cranial bones

5. the involuntary motion (motion we are not aware of) between the sacrum and the cranium.

Dr. Sutherland had study groups and his students taught my generation of students. As far as I know, Dr. Sutherland's original students have all passed on. It was an honor to have learned from his students in cranial courses and workshops.

I had the privilege to take courses with Dr. Ronald Becker, D.O. who was such a pure soul with an incredible ability to teach and heal.

I learned from Dr. Viola Frymann, D.O at cranial convocations. She also treated my son who had bronchitis and after one session he was cured.

There were many others whom I had the privilege to learn from and I feel very blessed to have had the time with these amazing mentors and teachers. These incredibly gifted teachers taught the next generation of teachers and the "life and breath" of cranial treatments live on.

Dr. Sutherland was the first to perceive subtly palpable movement within the bones of the cranium and went on to discover the continuity of this rhythmic fluid movement throughout all the tissues of the body.

Dr. Sutherland was able to feel this involuntary motion of the central nervous system which he called the Primary Respiratory Mechanism. It has its own rate per minute just as we have a heart rate and a respiratory rate. As an osteopath, I can feel this cranial motion and by feeling it I can treat and initiate a therapeutic response.

Cranial therapy can be used to treat anyone from infants to end of life patients. Treatment can restore motion, improve vitality (the ability to heal), and bring about a higher state of function.

I have had the opportunity to treat and correct a 3-month-old with sucking problems with a cranial treatment. I could describe this boy's head as misshapen and the back of his head pressed against the first vertebrae in his neck. The nerve (hypoglossal) that is involved with sucking was getting compressed because of the structural compression of the back of the head.

I treated and freed up all the bones, the dura of the cranium, and the rest of the body and within a few treatments, he was sucking strongly and efficiently instead of swallowing air and having to burp and be uncomfortable throughout his day.

Problems may begin with birth itself, often our first trauma, as an infant's head pushes through the birth canal. Some methods used by obstetricians such as forceps, vacuum extraction and Pitocin (to help speed labor) may add to the trauma and cause cranial distortions.

The head may not be shaped normally, and this may affect sucking, swallowing, colic, frequent spitting up, chronic ear infections and congestion, or even delayed development. Some problems such as learning disabilities, may not surface until a later date.

The cranial treatments use a gentle touch to feel the tissues and movement of the cranial mechanism. Many of my patients fall asleep during treatment and I leave them to sleep if they wish and move on to another treatment room.

I personally feel as though I am in a deep meditative state when I get treated. I also feel sensations in different parts of my body away from where the physician is placing his or her hands. I feel a fluid motion and a shift in my body. Usually, the pain I may be feeling is gone within a day of the treatment. My body responds very well to cranial treatments.

Craniosacral Therapy vs. Cranial Osteopathy?

Both therapies have their origins in Dr. Sutherland's work and because of Sutherland's background, became known as cranial osteopathy and only taught within osteopathic colleges.

Craniosacral therapists, by comparison, are not usually qualified osteopaths, dentists or M. D's that have taken the osteopathic cranial courses. Craniosacral therapists usually have taken courses at Upledger Institute.

Dr. John Upledger, D.O. was an osteopath who was willing to teach therapists outside the osteopathic realm such as massage therapists, physical therapists. and occupational therapists.

Dr. Sutherland's intention was to keep cranial therapy within the osteopathic realm as he himself was an osteopath and he stressed the importance of proficiency of anatomy and physiology before treating patients using cranial techniques. It does become a bit political and

I will leave it at that.

Osteopaths in the United States who are trained in cranial therapy, go to medical school just like their MD colleagues and continue on to residencies often side by side with their MD colleagues.

I personally feel working with lay people who learn cranial work without a foundation in anatomy, may be harmful to a patient.

If you are looking for a cranial osteopath to treat you in your area contact the Cranial Academy – www.cranialacademy.org, The Sutherland Cranial Teaching Foundation, www.sctf.com, or Biodynamic courses created by Dr. James Jealous, D.O.

www.osteodoc.com/biodynamics.htm

All of these courses require one to be a D.O., Dentist, or M.D. with full education of anatomy, structure, and function and a strong foundation in the cranial field.

CHAPTER 22

SELF-HELP GUIDE

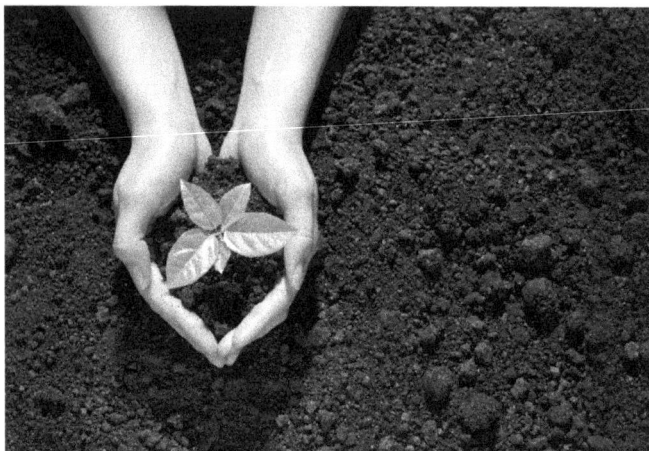

5 Steps to Improved Well-Being

1. What is "yoga breathing"?

Yoga breathing is a form of controlled deep breathing. Pranayama is a word used to describe the many breathing techniques used in yoga.

In Sanskrit, "prana" means energy, and "yama" means restrain or control. When we breathe in, we inhale oxygen, which our body needs to function. When we breathe out, we exhale carbon dioxide, a waste gas that our body doesn't need. Most of us take quick, shallow breaths, which don't benefit our body as much as deeper breaths.

Pranayama teaches you to breathe well, with an equal balance of nourishing oxygen inhaled and toxic carbon dioxide exhaled. It is important to focus on developing awareness of your breathing, rather than holding your breath. Breathing quickly and forcefully could make you feel faint, lightheaded and dizzy.

If you have asthma, heart disease or suffer from breathlessness, check with your doctor before beginning any yoga deep breathing techniques.

When you're practicing deep breathing, listen to your body. Keep your breath smooth and steady. Concentrate on slowly and calmly lengthening your out breath (exhalation), but don't feel that you have to breathe in or out for a certain period of time.

Yoga experts believe that deep breathing:

1. Improves the circulation of blood
2. Boosts the flow of oxygen that is supplied to your body
3. Assists your body to remove waste effectively.
4. Relaxes you and helps to reduce stress. What specific techniques can you try?

Think of the word "relax". It has two syllables, "re" and "lax". As you breathe in, think "re" to yourself, and as you breathe out, think "lax". Don't let your mind wander away from repeating the word "relax"' in tune with your breathing.

Or you can pick a two-syllable word that resonates with you.

When you breathe out, try to let go of any tensions in your body. Focus on the muscles that you know become tense when you're stressed.

Remember, every time you breathe out, "lax". The out-breath is the one to focus on, as the in-breath takes care of itself.

Or try counted breathing. As you breathe in, count slowly up to three or four, or whatever number seems comfortable for you. As you breathe out, count to three or four again. You may find that it's more comfortable to breathe in to a count of three and out to a count of four.

Try breathing in through your nose and out through your mouth. Keep your mouth very soft as you sigh the breath out. Breathe in through your nose, and out through your mouth. You may find it helpful to make a sound on the out-breath, such as "oooooh", or "aaaaah".

It might be challenging at first if you are not used to breathing from your abdomen.

When you breathe in, put your hands on your belly and breathe in through your nose as you expand your belly.

You then want to feel your ribs expand and then your chest expand.

When you breathe out, it's just the opposite: chest, ribs, and belly.

Think of it as pulling the navel towards the spine as you exhale. Take it slow and in time you will not need to think about what you are doing.

I take deep breaths in between patients if I am feeling stressed or just to practice when I am waiting in traffic or on line.

Proper breathing really helps slow down your nervous system and puts it into the rest and digest mode rather than the flight and fight mode.

2. Good posture

Be aware of how you are sitting and standing. The more bent over we are the less oxygen gets into our body and the less nourishment we get.

We also get more contracted as we age so it is important to stretch daily to open up your chest, allow your shoulders to relax and not stoop forward, and to lift up out of your pelvis and hips to avoid low back pain.

If you do not know where to begin, I recommend an Alexander Technique therapist to teach you about efficient posture and give you exercises to improve posture.

I also recommend going on YouTube and start doing restorative yoga to improve flexibility, which is gentle stretching with breath.

If you find areas of major restrictions such as the hips, low back, groin, chest, shoulders, and neck, I also recommend Yin Yoga which you can also find on YouTube. In Yin Yoga, you hold a posture for five minutes usually resting on props and pillows and breathing through the stretch.

You will feel very relaxed and restored after these postures.

3. Positive thinking and attitude of gratitude.

I recommend yoga nidra on YouTube. My favorite is Tripura yoga, the "Peace and Tranquility" video. I do this 1-hour guided visualization regularly in the morning and when I am finished I feel like a million dollars. My patients love it too.

Yoga nidra is a guided meditation which allows you to visualize areas of the body that are holding tension and releasing those areas of tension. In the beginning, you are guided to set an intention or goal.

Mine is always to stay balanced and not over do it, since that is my weakness. I tend to be the workaholic type, so I really need this guided meditation to have balance in my life. If I am over stressed,

BRIDGING THE GAP TO ONENESS

yoga nidra usually puts me back on the radar to balance and gives me a clearer focus on what really is important in my life.

4. Natural foods eaten calmly to half full capacity.

I always say eating foods from the ground and trees are the most healthy so fruits and vegetables, nuts, seeds, and beans, and grains – organic, of course.

We all metabolize differently. I have seen people on a macrobiotic diet who look frail and feel too weak while others thrive. The Paleo diet focuses on natural foods and protein. It follows a protocol of lots of fresh lean meats and fish, fruits, and vegetables, eggs, nuts and seeds as well as healthy oils, including olive and coconut oils.

You can't eat any processed foods on this diet and since our ancestors were hunter-gatherers, not farmers, say goodbye to wheat and dairy, along with other grains and legumes (such as peanuts and beans). Other foods to avoid:

- Dairy
- Refined sugar
- Potatoes
- Salt
- Refined vegetable oils, such as canola

I tend to lean towards this diet myself as I feel easily satisfied and don't have cravings and hunger. It is important to eat every 3-4 hours, so you do not get too hungry.

The vegans out there do well on more fats such as nuts, coconuts, avocado, hummus, tahini, beans, rice, and grains, but I feel the grains in general, if not eaten in moderation, can cause increased hunger and weight gain.

I had a patient who was vegan for years and she was very overweight as she ate too many grains. She had become diabetic and I told her it was time to turn toward chicken and fish and stop the grains and eat only quinoa. She basically went Paleo and became very thin and is no longer diabetic.

The most important issue I must stress is to stay away from hydrogenated fats, chemicals added to foods, white sugar, the excess of one glass of wine or a shot of liquor, excess coffee and avoid soda.

Try to start avoiding one unhealthy food or drink and when you are emotionally ready then add the next to avoid. Eventually, you will feel more satisfied with healthy eating and you will actually enjoy it.

5. Regular enjoyable exercise for 30 minutes for 4-5 times a week

When you are trying to heal it is important to not do any extreme exercise such as spinning, running fast, intense weight lifting or aerobics. These activities will add oxidative stress to your body and only make you feel weaker and depleted.

You must exercise in a balanced way with moderate types of exercise such as gentle yoga whether it is Hatha, Kundalini, restorative, Vinyasa flow, yin yoga or any of the other forms of yoga. Do not do Bikram or hot yoga when you are weak.

Other exercises that are beneficial are moderate walking in comfortable weather, swimming, stretching, light weights with more repetition 3 sets of 8 repetitions at the most. Treadmill or elliptical trainer walking only with a very light incline.

Do not push yourself to your limit and enjoy your workout.

Dancing of course is wonderful and can make you feel happy. All you need is music and a space to dance. It is a good idea to stretch after dancing as well.

I recommend to start exercising 3 days a week for a maximum of 30 minutes and work your way up to 5 to 6 days a week up to 1 hour. You must really listen now to when you feel like you are satisfied with the exercise and not get to a place of exhaustion.

Your goal and purpose is to heal not to burn yourself out. It might be a complete change from your previous days of high intensity workouts but now you are a new person and your needs are different.

You must listen to your body and what its limitations are, and you are the only one to know what they are. If you are doing a class do not look at the next person. Focus only on yourself. Once you accept your limitations gracefully you can start on your new path toward healing.

It is important to enjoy the exercise you chose so it can be an outlet for you as well as a productive part of your life.

Personally, exercise keeps me sane and gives me endurance and discipline. Since I started exercising at a young age, those endorphins we produce just make me feel great. I would at least recommend walking and stretching or restorative yoga as a minimum activity to clear the mind, burn some calories, and prevent osteoporosis.

There was a period in my life when my children were young that I had an overwhelming amount of responsibility as most parents do.

I took a 5-day break to take a JourneyDance™

certification course with founder, Toni Bergins. JourneyDance™ was just perfect for me as it was improvisational and explored all facets of emotions and creativity while dancing to music that ranged from African drumming, fluid, ethereal heart-warming, slow, fast, fun, and ener-gizing from withdrawing inward to adventuring outward.

The JourneyDance™ workshop also incorporated the chakras in the body to different styles of music. For example, if your power chakra or your third chakra was closed she would put on power-ful rhythmic music with her guidance for you to become powerful and strong within.

There were times when we cried, and times of laughter. We made collages from different maga-zine pictures which really opened up my creative side. As a mother of five boys, I needed this time to recharge. I first met Toni when she was teach-ing a class at The Kripalu Center for Yoga and Health in Stockbridge, Massachusetts.

I resonated with healing emotions through music and movement so much so that I went on to pursue training to become a JourneyDance™ facilitator.

Toni teaches others to become JourneyDance™ instructors as well as providing workshops and retreats. She travels around the world and teaches at various yoga centers. She also has retreats in the most beautiful places in the world such as Costa Rica and Jamaica, where you can feel freedom around you.

If you never had a chance to play as a child or if you enjoyed your childhood, this experience can really bring you back to all the joyful and most intimate times in your life.

JourneyDance™ allows you to feel your body, emotions and spirit using music with guided imagery, drama, the use of chakras, positive affirmations, getting in touch with your higher self, letting go of old patterns and finding health within.

For me personally, it allowed me to get in touch with my inner child and find true freedom and creativity within.

You can go on Toni's JourneyDance™ website: www.journeydance.com for more information.

There are many outlets that can express our creative side and we all must find one to break out of rigidity in our lives.

CHAPTER 23

SELF-HELP DETOX

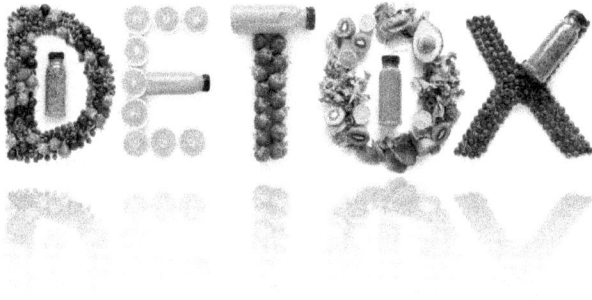

For those who do not eat healthy, or complain of recurrent gastrointestinal problems, food intolerances or sensitivity, chemical or environmental sensitivities, chronic headaches, skin conditions, muscle pain and fatigue and want to start on the right path toward healing.

I recommend a detox diet to cleanse physically from environmental toxins as well as an unhealthy diet.

The diet is low in lactose, sugar, fat, and gluten free. The goal is to cleanse the liver: the organ that detoxifies, to strengthen the absorption ability of the intestines, and to assist the colon to eliminate waste.

I recommend avoiding red meats, cold cuts, hot dogs, and sausages, canned meats, eggs, milk, cheese and all dairy, canned or creamed soups, coffee, tea, cocoa, alcoholic beverages, soda, sweet beverages, citrus, oat, spelt, Kamut, barley, amaranth, or gluten containing products, dried fruit, strawberries, margarine, shortening, unclarified butter, refined oils, peanuts, salad dressings, and spreads.

If you suffer from joint pain, I recommend that you do not eat nightshades such as potatoes, tomatoes, eggplant or bell peppers as they produce oxalic acid and may cause inflammation and joint pain.

So, what can you eat?

Chicken, turkey, lamb, all legumes, dried peas and lentils, cold water fish such a salmon, halibut, and mackerel. Legumes, seeds and peas contain lectins. Lectins are carbohydrate-binding proteins, macromolecules that are highly specific for sugar moieties of other molecules. Lectins on the outside of the legume, seed or pea may cause inflammation; I recommend that they are cooked in a pressure cooker to destroy the lectins if you have leaky gut or joint pain and arthritis.

Unsweetened live culture yogurt, rice milk, almond milk, and coconut milk, white or sweet potatoes, rice tapioca, buckwheat, millet, potato flour, arrowroot, gluten free products, homemade soups and broths. All vegetables preferably fresh, frozen or fresh juiced, fresh fruit, non-citrus herbal teas, cold expeller pressed unrefined flax, olive, sunflower oil, ghee, sesame oil, coconut oil. Pumpkin, squash, seeds, almonds, cashews, pecans and walnuts.

This detox is for 3 to 4 weeks. You are avoiding allergenic foods and eating whole foods that are not processed.

You should make sure to drink about 8 cups of water a day, preferably filtered.

Read labels carefully as well.

I recommend a detoxification powder preferably from pea protein or rice protein, like Pure Paleo-Cleanse Plus™ from Designs for Health®, or UltraClear® Renew from Metagenics®. They contain ingredients that support the liver and help with detoxification as well as cleansing both the intestines and colon.

You can look on my website **doctorbarbara.com** for the specific ingredients of these two products.

My patients tolerate this cleanse well, but you must keep in mind that if you have sugar cravings, other cravings or you have yeast over-growth in your gut then you may feel weak and even have diarrhea for the first few days until the body completely cleanses.

Once the cleanse is over, you can try to rotate

grains every three days (alternate spelt, oat, barley) but if you see that certain grains cause discomfort in your body it means that you should avoid that product.

The foods that I stay away from as much as possible are cheese, dairy, gluten, and sugar. Some people have many food sensitivities and need to be stricter. If you introduce a new food every week you can chart if there are any reactions.

Instant and Free Food Sensitivity Testing

Why is it so important to identify and avoid foods which we are sensitive to or can't tolerate? In a nutshell, food sensitivities equal stress and stress slows the metabolic rate, interferes with digestion and leads to a host of health issues.

Alternative medical practitioners utilize numerous approaches to determining if an individual is sensitive or allergic to a substance.

Common techniques include muscle testing and electrodermal biofeedback. All these approaches are based on the concept that the body exhibits a stress response when a substance is not right for the individual at that time.

Unfortunately, it can be pricey and time-consuming to get tested for food sensitivities by these practitioners. I'm excited to share with you an easy and FREE method for determining food sensitivities/allergies/intolerances at home!

This is NOT an exact science, but I believe it is a helpful tool. Know that the results of food sensitivity testing will depend on the mindset of the individual. If you think during the test, "I know I will be sensitive to this food and I hate that!" then it will most likely sway the test results.

Also, food sensitivities vary depending on the state of your digestive system. Are you angry and upset while doing this food sensitivity testing?

Anger actually slows digestion because it puts us into a sympathetic nervous system mode, instead of parasympathetic mode. So, the body senses the impaired digestion and this can manifest as being sensitive to more foods.

The Coca Pulse Test for Food Sensitivities, Allergies and Intolerances

Prestigious immunologist Dr. Arthur Coca published this test in 1956, and it provides an accessible way to trace a stress response to a certain food. It is based on the phenomena of how stress affects your pulse rate: if you are sensitive or allergic to a food, ingesting that food will immediately cause stress, which is manifested as an increased pulse rate.

Dr. Coca's book is now public domain and available free on the internet. He directs you to record your diet for 5-7 days and record your pulse 14 times per day (before rising, before retiring, before each meal and at 30-minute intervals after each meal).

If you eat a food you are allergic/sensitive to, you will calculate a quickened pulse after the meal at which you ate it. Then, you can analyze your food journal with the recorded pulses and determine the foods to which you react.

Although the Coca Pulse test is free (no pricey food intolerance lab tests), it is a bit time consuming and it can be hard to remember when to take your pulse. I prefer The LNT Coca Pulse Test.

The LNT Coca Pulse Test for Food Sensitivities

This is a modified version of the Pulse Test that I find quicker, easier and altogether preferable. I learned this tool as part of the curriculum at the Nutritional Therapy Association.

"LNT" stands for Lingual-Neural Testing, which utilizes the communication pathways between the mouth and the central nervous system. Simply tasting a food sends messages throughout the body, and the body will communicate through a quickened pulse if this food is not ideal for you.

This version of the pulse test allows you specifically to test one food at a time and immediately learn if the food is beneficial or stressful to your body. It is like the instant- gratification method of Dr. Coca's original test.

Do this test 1-2 hours after eating or drinking anything. Start when you are mentally, emotionally and physically relaxed. Always take your pulse for one full minute – don't take it for 30 seconds and multiply it by two.

While sitting, take a deep breath and slowly exhale. Take your pulse by counting how many times your heart beats in one exact minute. It may be easiest to feel your pulse by placing two fingers on the upper right side of your neck. Record this pulse rate.

Next, put a piece of the food in question in your mouth. It is okay to chew, but don't swallow. Taste the food for at least 30 seconds. Then, take your pulse again for a full minute with the food in your mouth. Spit out the food and rinse your mouth with filtered water.

If the pulse rate rises 6 or more points with a food, it indicates a stress reaction and that food should be avoided. Remember, food sensitivities can heal through diet and lifestyle changes, so it will be possible to re-test and reintroduce these foods after a period of healing.

Let the pulse return to the baseline before testing with a different food.

NOTE: If testing eggs, test the egg yolk and the

egg white separately. Egg yolks are often better tolerated than egg whites.

Food sensitivities aren't necessarily permanent.

Food sensitivities and even some food allergies can heal with time and a nourishing diet. Food sensitivities occur because the lining of our intestine is permeated with small holes, allowing undigested proteins or partially-digested food particles to escape into the bloodstream. This triggers antibodies to attack the foreign particles in the blood. This is called leaky gut.

Sometimes when addressing a food sensitivity, all it requires is temporarily eliminating the food in question for a few months. Re-test the foods at intervals of 3 months to see if you can re-introduce them.

In more serious cases, a comprehensive protocol may be required to seal up the leaky gut, so the food can be ingested without triggering those antibodies.

The GAPS diet is an excellent tool for this and is outlined in *The Gut and Psychology Syndrome Diet* book. Another powerful protocol is the Autoimmune Paleo Protocol, outlined in *The Paleo Approach* book.

Have you been tested for food sensitivities? Have you noticed a difference when you avoid eating foods to which you are sensitive?

I find that most people who have food sensitivities have "burnt out adrenals" from pushing too hard in life so it is so important to really look into stressors, emotional imbalances and spirit imbalances that may have caused these food sensitivities.

I tell my patients that they have to work on letting go of control and start finding balance in their lives... not to push too hard, create down time for yourself, meditate, gentle yoga, at least 7-8 hours of sleep and listening to your body. The truth is this is the hardest part of the detox diet as it requires you to make permanent changes in your life style.

I had a patient that suffered from severe constipation and was doing the GAPS diet and eating broths with bone marrow and fish bones and it was helping a bit but what helped her the most was The Journey™ by Brandon Bays. She ended up becoming a Journey Facilitator by taking courses with Brandon Bays.

The human individual is so complex, unlike a car. There are so many layers to unravel and what works for one person may not work for the next. We must keep trying to find our path from within and finding the right healers to facilitate this process.

In my work as a physician, I try to be an advocate for patients. I see what tests were not ordered, and what conventional doctors did not address. I look between the cracks and find out the root of the problem. Sometimes it is easy and sometimes it is a drawn-out process but as healers, we work as a team to find health within.

CHAPTER 24

VITAMINS

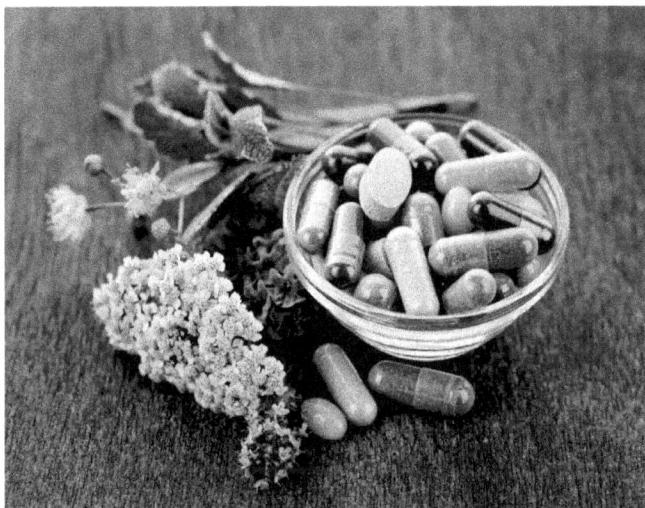

What vitamins may be beneficial? I recommend that all patients feeling depleted, stressed, and anxious check for Vitamin B12, folate, homocysteine, 25-hydroxyvitamin D, 1-25 dihydroxy vitamin D and MTHFR genetic blood testing along with their routine labs.

B12 deficiency can cause fatigue which is the most common symptom of people who have low levels of vitamin B12. But fatigue by itself can be a sign of almost any health condition – or just that you haven't been sleeping enough! Other signs of B12 deficiency include weight loss, constipation or diarrhea, nausea and vomiting, abdominal bloating and gas, numbness or tingling in the hands and feet, loss of balance, and a sore, red tongue.

Folate deficiency – Isolated folate deficiency is uncommon; it usually coexists with other nutrient deficiencies because of its strong association with poor diet, alcoholism, and, sometimes, malabsorption disorders.

Megaloblastic anemia, which is characterized by large, abnormally nucleated erythrocytes, is the primary clinical sign of a deficiency of folate or vitamin B12.

Symptoms of megaloblastic anemia include weakness, fatigue, difficulty concentrating, irritability, headache, heart palpitations, and shortness of breath.

Folate deficiency can also produce soreness and shallow ulcerations in the tongue and oral mucosa; changes in skin, hair, or fingernail pigmentation; and elevated blood concentrations of homocysteine.

Elevated levels of homocysteine is a high-risk factor for coronary artery disease. Women with insufficient folate intakes are at increased risk of giving birth to infants with neural tube defects. Inadequate maternal folate status has also been associated with low infant birth weight, preterm delivery, and fetal growth retardation.

Researchers have pointed out that increasing

levels of vitamin D among the general population could prevent chronic diseases that claim nearly one million lives throughout the world each year. Studies have shown that if you improve your vitamin D status, it reduces risk of colorectal cancer, prostate cancer, and a whole host of other deadly cancers by 30 to 50 percent.

Vitamin D also fights infections, including colds and the flu, as it regulates the expression of genes that influence your immune system to attack and destroy bacteria and viruses and is very important for reducing hypertension, atherosclerotic heart disease, heart attack, and stroke.

Vitamin D is also a potent immune modulator, making it very important for the prevention of autoimmune diseases, like multiple sclerosis and inflammatory bowel disease.

However, serum vitamin 25-hydroxyvitamin D is not an entirely accurate indicator of vitamin D status. According to the new research long term use of vitamin D may promote atherosclerosis (hardening of the arteries) or kidney stones. In Dr. Alan R. Gaby's book, *Nutritional Medicine* (www.doctorgaby.com), he does not recommend more than 2,000 units of vitamin D unless someone has prostate cancer, malabsorption issues, or drug induced vitamin D deficiency. The Vitamin 25-hydroxyvitamin D levels vary among populations, sun exposure, age, body mass index, skin color so therefore, the potential benefits must outweigh the potential risks. Vitamin D from sunlight is recommended for those who do not have risk factors for about 5-15 minutes three times a week to the arms, legs, and face between 10 am and 3 pm during the Spring, Summer, and Fall seasons. Vitamin 1-25 dihydroxyvitamin D can be low in kidney disease and high in parathyroid disease, lymphoma, and sarcoidosis the vitamin D dosing is somewhat controversial as you have just read. It is a benefit versus risk situation.

MTHFR

All humans have the same set of genes, but differences come from the tiny *variations* in those genes. One of the more common and potentially dangerous variations is known as an MTHFR mutation.

This gene variation can impact how well your body metabolizes folate and folic acid. Both are forms of vitamin B9, required for numerous critical bodily functions. Unfortunately, a fault in this metabolic cycle is linked to many serious health problems

Symptoms of MTHFR

There are many different symptoms someone with one or both gene mutations might encounter. Not everyone has the same set of symptoms because there are many other genetic and environmental differences that complicate health.

Nevertheless, if you boil it down, there is a key systemic problem that comes from low methylation and it causes three different symptom areas.

Systemic Problems

Homocysteine levels are too high because not enough methylfolate is available to convert the homocysteine into methionine. High homocysteine levels are often blamed for cardiovascular events like strokes and heart attacks. In addition, without methylfolate, SAMe and Glutathione in the body are often low (these are responsible for serotonin production and detoxification respectively).

Basically, you can think of methylfolate (L-MTHF or 5-MTHF) as being able to convert the bad guy (Homocysteine) into something good for the body (Methionine) as well as promote the good guys (SAMe and Glutathione) responsible for neurotransmitter balance and helping rid your body of heavy metals, environmental toxins, etc.

Three Symptom Areas:

1. Central Nervous System disorders – some of these come from not having enough SAMe. SAMe is responsible for creating Serotonin and neurotransmitters responsible for mood, motivation,

and to some degree energy levels. If these neuro-transmitters are low, then depression is often the result, but even aggression and alcoholism are symptoms sometimes found in men. Pregnant women may encounter extreme postpartum depression.

In addition, illnesses like Fibromyalgia, Chronic Fatigue Syndrome, Migraines, IBS (Irritable Bowel Syndrome), Memory loss with Alzheimer's and Dementia as well as other psychiatric problems can be tied to this issue (OCD, Bipolar, Schizophrenia, and more).

2. Cardiovascular problems often occur when Homocysteine levels in the body are too high.

Heart attack, Stroke, Blood clots, Peripheral neuropathy, Anemia even Miscarriages, and Congenital birth defects can be related to this issue among other symptoms.

3. Environmental poisoning can increase when not enough Glutathione is present to detox the body. Glutathione is responsible for detoxifying the body of heavy metals, and toxins that we encounter in the environment. Glutathione is our body's most powerful antioxidant.

When a body gets too burdened by heavy metals and toxins, a lot of unexpected health problems emerge.

Some symptoms of this can be: nausea, diarrhea,

abdominal pain, liver and kidney dysfunction, hypertension, tachycardia, pulmonary fibrosis, asthma, immune problems, hair loss, rashes and much more.

As I was writing this book a nutritional supplement company representative came to my office with some new products and one such product is liposomal glutathione. Glutathione taken by mouth as a pill will not be effective as an antioxidant because the gut flora will inactivate it. So, one can take N-acetylcysteine (NAC) as this will break down in the liver to Glutathione.

Most glutathione supplements on the market do not use Acetyl-L-Glutathione, and you are only absorbing between 1 and 3 percent of their value. Essentially throwing your money out the window. Acetyl-L-Glutathione has an absorption rate of over 90 percent, allowing your body to use it to its full effect.

Acetyl-L-glutathione is a supplement formulated to withstand the gut environment improving the absorption and bioavailability of this antioxidant.

I personally started using liposomal glutathione formulated with sunflower oil. It is absorbed under the tongue directly going systemically into the bloodstream through the saliva.

This liposomal glutathione changed my life in just 2 weeks. I am now sleeping 2 hours less per night which has been my biggest test over the past 15 years. I have the genetic heterozygous gene that does not metabolize folic acid into methylfolate. Methylfolate supports methylation which in turn supports cell growth and division.

Glutathione amounts need to be high enough in your system in order to methylate folic acid or one can get side effects from methylfolate. It is also important to drink enough electrolytes to support methylation or you can get side effects of too much methylfolate in your system such as muscle spasm, dizziness, urinary frequency, and nausea.

After this nutritional supplement company representative came into my office I decided that I must start on a regimen that I suggest to my patients. Doctors can sometimes make the worst patients. I put together vitamins that were appropriate for me including methylfolate, B12, borage oil and liposomal glutathione and drank a good electrolyte formula and water.

A miracle occurred for me within 2 weeks and the 12-hour sleep requirement was reduced by 2 hours. I am sure within 6 months my new 10-hour sleep requirement will be further reduced. I am now embarking on decreasing medication and my goal is to be off all medication that was originally used for extreme insomnia and anxiety/depression from low serotonin.

I am very excited about my new freedom of

needing less sleep and having more time in the day to enjoy life and to be more productive. We should all merit to have complete healing and I am so appreciative for this gift of liposomal glutathione. For more information on Phase 2 glutathione conjugation, I recommend that you check out:

http://www.herbaltransitions.com/ GlutathioneConjugation.html.

Multiple Cause Disorders

Sometimes diseases/disorders fall under a 'multiple-pronged' cause, meaning the causes of it stem from genetic, environmental, microbial and/or bacterial problems. Autism is a big one that falls into a 'two-pronged' cause category along with Fibromyalgia, Chronic Fatigue Syndrome, Lyme Disease and more. MTHFR is at the top of a list of 16 genetic defects for Autism.

One study showed 98% of children with Autism had one or both MTHFR gene defects and a clinical study indicated that mothers with MTHFR who didn't take folate during pregnancy were 7 times more likely to have an autistic child than mothers without the MTHFR gene defect. Colon and gastric cancers also have key links to the MTHFR gene defects.

I recommend that if there is a MTHFR genetic defect in one or two genes then I would give

Methyl Folate 5 mg to 15 mg a day depending on age, weight and symptoms with Vitamin B12 1000ug a day to an adult. I would start on low doses of methyl folate to make sure the patient does not experience side effects and stops the regimen. I recommend the site MTHFR.net for more information about starting on methylfolate.

I often recommend in fish oils (EPA/DHA) for their benefits which include an ability to aid in the treatment of various heart diseases, high cholesterol, depression, anxiety, ADHD, weakened immune system, cancer, diabetes, inflammation, arthritis, irritable bowel disorder, AIDS, Alzheimer's disease, eye disorders, macular degeneration and ulcers.

Fish oils also aid weight loss, healthy pregnancy, fertility and skin care (particularly for conditions such as psoriasis and acne).

Most of the health benefits of fish oil can be attributed to the presence of omega-3 essential fatty acids like Docosahexaenoic acid (DHA) and Eicosapentaenoic acid (EPA). Other useful essential fatty acids in fish oil include Alpha- linolenic acid or ALA and Gamma-linolenic acid or GLA.

In the past 10 years, many Americans have turned to omega-3 fish oil supplements, which have benefits for healthy people and also those with heart disease.

Omega-3 fatty acids may help to:

- Lower blood pressure and reduce triglycerides
- Slow the development of plaque in the arteries
- Reduce the chance of abnormal heart rhythm
- Reduce the likelihood of heart attack and stroke
- Lessen the chance of sudden cardiac death in people with heart disease

The American Heart Association (AHA) recommends that everyone eats fish (particularly fatty, cold-water fish) at least twice a week. Salmon, mackerel, herring, sardines, lake trout, and tuna are especially high in omega-3 fatty acids. While foods are your best bet for getting omega-3s in your diet, fish oil supplements are also available for those who do not like fish.

How much omega-3 fish oil is safe?

The AHA says taking up to 3 grams of fish oil daily in supplement form is considered safe. Don't take more than that unless you discuss it with your doctor first.

Side effects from omega-3 fish oil may include:

- A fishy taste in your mouth
- Fishy breath
- Stomach upset
- Loose stools
- Nausea

Taking more than 3 grams of fish oil daily may increase the risk of bleeding.

I tell my patients to freeze the fish oil capsule if they are experiencing fishy breath or stomach upset.

I also recommend a good multivitamin with iron for menstruating women, and if you have a stressed lifestyle and are not eating as well as you should. I recommend a multivitamin without iron if iron levels are normal as excess of iron can increase the risk of heart disease.

It is important to look at vitamin labels and make sure there are no fillers, artificial colors and additives.

I have many patients taking many antioxidants, and herbs for their conditions. It is very important to know if the vitamin or herb does not interfere with medications one is taking as well as the possible side effects of the supplements.

I prefer liquid or powder over capsules or pills for better absorption in the digestive tract.

I tell my patients who are suffering from cardio-vascular disease or who have a predisposition and those patients who have a family history of cancer to also take antioxidants such as: Turmeric (curcumin), grape seed extract, pycnogenol, vitamin E 400IU-800IU, selenium 200ug - 400 ug, Vit A 25,000IU, B-Carotene 25,000IU, Vitamin C 1000mg-3000mg, to name a few.

I also recommend probiotics taken once a day to replenish good bacteria in our gut especially if we are on antibiotics, steroids, birth control pills or under a lot of stress. One should take the probiotic or homemade yogurt 2 hours away from the medication so as not to diminish the action of the medication.

I would advise to have a proper evaluation for the supplements that would be right for your individual needs.

Diet is very important and of course requires the most discipline which is not always so easy, but once you are feeling healthier and stronger your diet becomes your way of life.

CHAPTER 25

LIFE GOALS

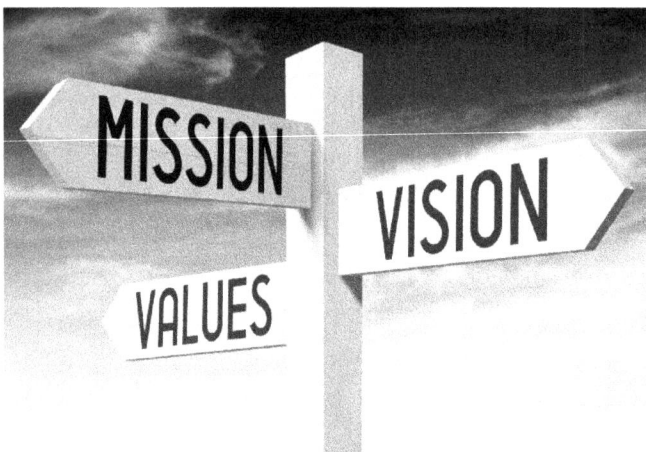

We are all trying to find health in life – whether it is physically, emotionally, or spiritually.

There are only a few moments of bliss when we are in an amazing place or on a natural high from life. The rest is hard work and if you have the right attitude you will grow in your journey towards health and wellness.

We all need to have personal dreams of where we want to be in life and through our dreams and actions, we can succeed. On the road towards success, there may be obstacles along the way and you must listen to those obstacles.

I admit as a young and active girl I did not listen to my obstacles and thought I was limitless until I finally hit the wall and got the message to change. I cannot go back and change the past, but I can change the present and have dreams for the future. There were no mistakes as I changed and grew from the challenges I faced.

I remember when I first arrived in Israel at age 21. My heart and soul were in love with the land and I said to myself while standing overlooking the Old City of Jerusalem, that I would be back one day in the future – without question. This affirmation did come true as it was my longing.

I married a man who also wanted to live in Israel as that was very important to me. It took us 26 years to finally make it to Israel as we both felt ties to our families and our parents.

We always had our plans to go: our 2-year plans, 5-year plans and then one day the door opened for us after my mother passed away.

My father had two strokes, my youngest son was going into high school and all my other sons were grown up. I looked at my husband and said if not now – when? He said I was right and we proceeded with the process to live in Israel. My father came with us and we were blessed as my dad now lives with us with a caretaker that is affordable, and our dreams have come true.

I've had other goals that I pursued, and some

worked, and some didn't as ultimately, we are not in control, but we do have to try and do the work.

Then there are the times when you don't plan, and life just happens. You can see the higher force present in your life. For me, it was having children. I was not raised in a large family and was very career oriented. I had five boys, two while in residency.

I was clueless but yes, I learned instinctively how to be a mother as well as reading about raising children and having role models around me in my community. Little did I know I was going to have five boys. I told my husband I was not maternal before I married him. I can now laugh about it.

Over ten years ago, I began writing this book as part of a goal to document my journey and offer my perspective on healing. I had a patient who was an editor and she offered her assistance. About a quarter way through the editing, her workload at her job prevented her from completing the project. As the same time, my busy practice and family life put this goal on hold. The timing was not right, so I let it go.

I saved everything and over one year ago I randomly asked a supplement representative who came into my office if he knew someone who is an editor and he mentioned his wife. We met on the phone and began to connect regularly via phone and Skype to begin the journey of writing this book.

The timing was finally right, and this book just flowed from there. Life can be random at times and fluid as well, like the waves of an ocean. Sometimes you just need to be still and allow the life force to flow through you, as Dr. Sutherland would say.

I hope you find this book helpful in assisting you towards your optimal health.

If you need more assistance you can go to my website: **www.doctorbarbara.com** and schedule an appointment for me to be your health advocate and guide in your process toward optimal health.

IN CONCLUSION

One such case that I remember was a woman who had suffered from fibromyalgia, difficulty swallowing, reflux, and phlebitis (clots in her legs) during all her pregnancies. She was unhappily married but did not mention this to me during her first visit.

I gave her Vitamin C and multivitamin IV drips to improve her immune system and I treated her with cranial treatments to help her pain and help her release her tension and emotions. She had done all these studies on her swallowing difficulties at a specialty hospital on this disorder. She was given medications but without relief. She lived on liquid and purified foods only.

I mentioned to her that difficulty swallowing has to do with the 6th chakra which relates to using her voice in communication. I gave her yoga exercises to strengthen her throat and her emotions about communicating.

She admitted to me she was scared to divorce her husband who was cruel and abusive. Why? He was wealthy, and she thought her family would think she was crazy to divorce a wealthy man. She eventually developed her inner strength and told her husband she wanted a divorce. She made that crucial decision and her swallowing problems subsided completely and eventually she remarried and became a massage therapist.

Another case involved a woman I diagnosed with fibromyalgia and Hepatitis C just a few weeks before her marriage in 1996. She was a high-powered woman who worked for a prestigious NY magazine and was an emergency room nurse. She did not know what rest meant.

She lived a NYC lifestyle working and was partying hard as a single woman. She had a history of being an alcoholic but became sober two years before she married and became an AA (Alcohol Anonymous) sponsor.

When I initially saw this patient, she collapsed with exhaustion and body pain. She had a very lengthy medical history including hemorrhaging during labor. The patient survived the crisis after several blood transfusions, however her child did not survive. She spent many years grieving over the loss of her child. She had multiple complaints such as recurrent sinusitis, body pain, numbness, radiating pain down her arm, hip bursitis, ear infections, and a sluggish thyroid.

As sick as she was she was unable to get long-term disability due to her Hepatitis C and history of alcoholism even though she had been sober for two years. The disability case put a lot of stress on the patient as she had to stop working and rely on her husband and the universe financially.

Her mantra was "let go or be dragged". This patient was diagnosed with Hepatitis C after her labs revealed elevated liver enzymes. I made this diagnosis because she had blood transfusions which were not screened in the 1980's. She was started on medication to cure the hepatitis C by her gastroenterologist. She was cured of this illness. Unfortunately, she had side effects such as medication induced psychosis, frequent infections, bone loss of her jaw and osteoarthritis of her neck, low back and knees.

Her gastroenterologist that treated her for the Hepatitis C was not very helpful and told her to stop the treatment after 8 months but did not offer her support.

I worked with this patient from head to toe. I first

started her on medication for the psychosis which finally resolved within 2 months of stopping the medication for the Hepatitis C. I treated her using osteopathy, IV vitamin drips, and acupressure. She had severe nerve pain in her mouth from the bone loss that breathing in air was a painful sensation.

She desperately needed to see a dentist to remove her teeth and replace them with

implants and bridges. The dental work she needed was not affordable in the USA, so she traveled to Costa Rica for this undertaking.

Her immune system weakened further, and she ended up with bacterial meningitis and somehow survived after being hospitalized in a coma with a high fever of 104. I helped guide her husband to get her to the hospital ASAP. He was on his way to NYC for a band rehearsal as his wife was getting sicker and I told him to turn around and get her into a hospital, hydrated and treated.

I remember I was about to go to sleep as I was leaving to take my Osteopathic boards in Dallas Texas the next day. We stayed in contact before and after my board exams and she survived meningitis but then had sequelae of headaches, light sensitivity, and cognitive problems. She had a ten-year process of recovery. I told her to get enough rest and take the pressure off herself.

We worked together on her dynamics with her

father and siblings as a child and on letting go of old habits from her childhood that would be detrimental to her in her healing. Her father used to push her hard to always be productive and now she needed to rest and gain her strength back.

She really learned to let go of pushing herself even though she still would fall back into old patterns from time to time. In those 10 years she had a complete knee replacement, fractured left ankle, reflex sympathetic dystrophy (RSD is continual pain and numbness from increased sympathetic stimulation in an area of the body usually after surgery or trauma), degenerative disc disease and arthritis of her low back and neck with frequent nerve blocks to break the pain cycle. At one point when she had severe pain from her teeth she was on painkillers. Once her teeth were restored she decided to get off the pain medications and went to a hospital to detox off the medications. I was supportive of her process but also concerned for her. She went through hell for a few weeks detoxing.

Eventually, within time and treatments, her immune system became stronger and she was able to start working again although with a different mindset. She was voted "most changed" by the prestigious magazine reunion she attended.

This patient strived to improve her health by creating balance, exercising, resting, guided imagery relaxation, improving her diet, consistent osteopathic treatments, intravenous vitamin treatments, and acupressure.

She also read Dr. Sarno's book and started to journal her anger as well as intensive therapy for post-traumatic stress. I was an advocate and a physician/healer in her process of regaining health.

She is now out of the woods, but she has to maintain her newfound lifestyle. Her positive attitude, incredible inner strength, and compliance (most of the time) helped her to heal.

We never gave up! She still has arthritis and bone loss, but she rarely gets infections now. We are all a work in progress some more than others and this is the journey of life.

I have had many instances where I needed to guide patients into making lifestyle changes in order to improve their health. I had one patient who was raising one child with special needs and the other with a chronic illness all while teaching high intensity spin classes, aerobics and lifting weights. She was exhausted and was unable to lose weight no matter how hard she tried.

I told her that her adrenals were producing a lot of cortisol and that she would burn out if she continued at her pace. The increased cortisol production from stress would not let her shed pounds. She was also low in testosterone.

I started her on bio-identical hormones and I encouraged her to do more gentle yoga and less heavy workouts and instead to walk. She eventually became a yoga instructor, slowed down her pace, lost inches and felt great.

I have encouraged patients to make lifestyle including career changes. I have seen patients completely heal after changing their career path and becoming fulfilled.

Our health is linked to how we feel about ourselves and our inner power. Once these patients changed careers they had more inner peace and led happier healthier lives.

I try to empower my patients to make the changes they need in order for them to find that balance within and to reach their optimal health.

We are all on a journey and ultimately it is all about how we respond to stress in our lives. Simple tools to keep us balanced are to pray, meditate and breathe deeply.

We need to try to always see the glass half full and change any negative thought patterns when they occur but to also be in touch with our emotions and feel the pain and then to let it go. We need to be fluid with change and for some of us this is very hard to do.

That is why meditation and prayer are important in our daily lives.

We should spend at least thirty minutes daily filling up our vessel with exercise, meditation, reading, and any constructive activity that nourishes our being. We are not just humans doing but human beings.

Sometimes we need to be still and listen and at other times we need to take action but not be attached to the outcome. You can't always get what you want but you do get what you need.

What I am saying is very hard to put into action but with discipline, consciousness, meditation and guidance we can apply these principles to our daily lives. We may fall at first and repeat our past mistakes but after a while we will get the hang of it.

If we are tested with health issues we need to pursue and take action and walk on the bridge to vitality and healing.

Healing may take work and we must not be passive about it and let all the decisions be made by our medical doctors.

We need objective advocates to help guide us on our path toward healing with a body, mind, spirit approach. Sometimes we need to come to acceptance and inner peace with our situation and be patient with time and effort to gain our health and vitality.

The more open minded you are about all the

modalities for healing the better off you are. Sometimes western medicine is the answer and sometimes not or it's a combination of both or neither.

The purpose of this book is to help guide you toward your true vitality and health and for you to gain wisdom along the way and find peace within yourself.

I am more than happy to help guide you to improved health, vitality and inner peace.

This is my mission!

~ Dr. Barbara

Excerpt from a patient: *"Dr. Barbara, just a note to say that I am at long last feeling a sense of acceptance and calm and crawling out of the cage with confidence and strength and credit the fact that I have you as my guide".*

MY FAVORITE RESOURCES

<u>**BOOKS:**</u>

Nutrition

1. *Grain Brain*, by David Perlmutter, MD

2. *Prescription for Nutritional Healing, Fifth Edition: A Practical A-to-Z Reference to Drug-Free Remedies Using Vitamins, Minerals, Herbs & Food*, by Phyllis A. Balch CNC

3. *Milk the Deadly Poison*, by Robert Cohen

4. *Breaking the Vicious Cycle*, by Elaine Gloria Gottschall/ Rochel Weiss

5. *Adrenal Fatigue: The 21st Century Stress Syndrome*, by James L. Wilson MD, DC, PHD

6. *Nutritional Medicine*, by Alan R. Gaby, MD

7. *Hypothyroidism: The Unsuspected Illness*, by Broda Barnes

8. *Stay Young & Sexy with Bio-Identical Hormone Replacement*, by Jonathan V. Wright, MD

9. *Wilson's Syndrome, The Miracle of Feeling Well*, by Denis E. Wilson, MD

10. *Women's Bodies, Women's Wisdom*, by Christiane Northrup, MD

11. *The Wisdom of Menopause*, by Christiane Northrup, MD

Homeopathy

12. *Everybody's Guide to Homeopathic Medicines* third revised edition of the most popular family homeopathic guidebook in the world, teaches step-by-step

how to select the correct homeopathic remedy for numerous common ailments and injuries, originally published in1984. Authors: Dana Ullman & Stephen Cummings

Ayurveda

13. *Perfect Health*, by Deepak Chopra, MD

14. *Ayurvedic Cooking for Self-Healing*, by Usha Lad & Vasant Lad

15. *Prakriti: Your Ayurvedic Constitution*, by Dr. Robert Svoboda

16. *Yoga & Ayurveda: Self-Healing and Self-Realization*, Paperback – by David Dr. Frawley

Medicine and Osteopathy

17. *Life in Motion*, by Rollin E. Becker, DO

18. *The Heart of Listening I* and *II*, by Hugh Milne, DO

19. *Touch of Life*, by Dr. Fulford

20. *Philosophy of Osteopathy, Philosophy and Mechanical Principles of Osteopathy*. Can be purchased online: academyofosteopathy.org

21. *Think Away Your Pain*, *The Mind-Body Journal*, DVD and CD, and *The Mindbody Workbook for Journaling*, by Dr. David Schechter, MD

22. A *Mind of Your Own*, by Kelly Brogan, MD and Co-Author - Integrative Therapies for Depression

23. *What Your Doctor May Not Tell You about Depression* and *The Breakthrough Integrative Approach for Effective Treatment*, by Michael Schachter, MD

24. *The Prostate Cancer Revolution*, Robert Bard, MD

25. *Psychology and Mind Body Spirit Methodologies PTSD The Body Keeps the Score*, by Bessel Van der Kolk, MD

26. *The Journey, A Practical Guide to Healing* and *Living The Journey*, by Brandon Bays

27. *The Book of Chakra Healing*, by Liz Simpson

28. HayHouse.com founded by Louise Hay the forerunner of body/mind/spirit empowerment

29. *Healing Back Pain / The Mindbody Prescription* DVD by John E. Sarno, MD, available on Dr. Sarno's website.

30. *The Mindbody Prescription Healing the Body Healing the Pain*, by John E. Sarno, MD

31. *The Divided Mind*, By John E. Sarno, MD

32. *Spontaneous Healing*, by Andrew Weil, MD Chapter 2 of the book discusses Dr. Andrew Weil observing Dr Fulford, DO, healing patients. www.drweil.com

33. JourneyDance™ workshops and classes - Toni Bergins, www.journeydance.com

Acupuncture

34. *Traditional Acupuncture: The Law of the Five Elements*, by Dianne M. Connelly, DC, PhD.

35. *Healing Your Emotions; Discover your Five Element Type and Change Your Life*, by Angela Hicks and John Hicks.

36. *Staying Healthy with the Seasons*, by Elson M. Haas, MD

Supplements and Herbs

37. Designs for Health Supplements
38. Metagenics supplements
39. Pure Encapsulations supplements
40. Gaia Herbs
41. Emerson Ecologics distributing company

Yoga and Meditation

42. The Kripalu Yoga Collection DVD, *Gentle Yoga*, by Jurian Hughes
43. *Deep and Delicious Yoga*, by Jurian Hughes
44. myyogaworks.com website for beginners to advanced classes
45. *Deep Relaxation: Divine Sleep Yoga Nidra*, Audio CD and MP3 Download, by Jennifer Reis
46. *Yoga: The Spirit and Practice of Moving into Stillness*, by Erich Schiffman and Trish O'Reilly
47. *Tripura Yoga Peace and Tranquility* - Yoga Nidra guided meditation on YouTube
48. *Restorative Yoga Practice; Gentle Beginners Sessions with Deborah Donohue*, DVD
49. *Natural Birth Secrets: An Insider's Guide How To Give Birth Holistically, Healthfully and Safely, and Love the Experience*, by Anne Margolis CNM, MSN
50. *Trauma Release Formula: The Revolutionary Step by Step Program for Eliminating Effects of Childhood Abuse, Trauma, Emotional Pain and Crippling Inner Stress, to Living in Joy without Drugs or Therapy*, by Anne Margolis, CNM, MSN
http://homesweethomebirth.com

Breathwork

51. *Breathe Deep, Laugh Loudly*, by Judith Kravitz

52. *The Breathing Book*, by Donna Farhi

53. *The Hindu Yogi Science of the Breath*, by Yogi Ramacharaka

54. *Breathing*, by Michael Sky

55. *Oxygen Healing Therapies*, Nathaniel Altman

56. *The Karma of Materialism*, by Rudolf Steiner

57. Transformational Breath Foundation - www.breath2000.com
e-mail: info@breath2000.com

COMPOUNDING PHARMACIES

Rye Beach Pharmacy
Rye, NY
www.ryerx.com

Apple Valley Pharmacy
Goshen, NY
www.applevalleypharmacy.com

Life Science Pharmacy
Harriman, NY
www.lifesciencepharmacy.com

Millers Pharmacy
Wyckoff NJ
www.millerspharmacy.com

Women's International Pharmacy
Madison, Wisconsin
www.womensinternational.com

Medaus Pharmacy
Birmingham, AL
www.medaus.com

SPECIALTY LABORATORIES

IGeneX, Inc
Lyme Testing and Lyme Related Testing
www.igenex.com

Genova Labs
Nutritional Analysis, Stool Analysis for Parasites,
Candida and Bacteria, Saliva Hormone Panel
www.gdx.net

ABOUT THE AUTHOR

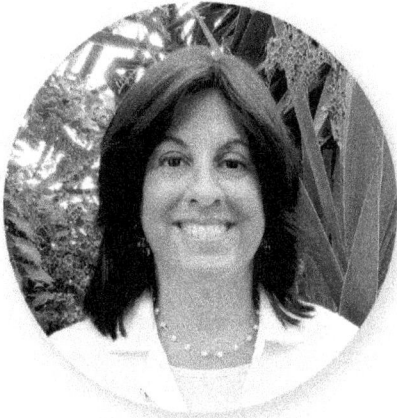

Doctor Barbara is an Osteopathic Physician, with a focus on Family Medicine and Integrative Medicine for over 25 years. Doctor Barbara has dedicated her practice to treating the whole person, focusing on the cause of imbalance rather than treating just symptoms.

She is an innovative and caring practitioner whose philosophy is to empower her patients to make lifestyle changes that promote healing at the level of the body, mind and spirit. Doctor Barbara is certified in Yoga and JourneyDance™. She incorporates Movement Therapy in her practice.

Doctor Barbara is New York State licensed and Board certified in Family Medicine and Osteopathic Manipulative Medicine. She is a Graduate of the New York College of Osteopathic Medicine. She is certified in Botox˚ Cosmetics and Dermal Fillers. Her years of training in Cranial Therapy, Osteopathic Manipulative Medicine and Trigger Point Injections enable her to be very sensitive and creative in the Art of Facial Rejuvenation. Doctor Barbara lectures in the Tri-State area on Women's Health, Bioidentical Hormones, Integrative Medicine, Osteopathy and the Art and Science of Cosmetic rejuvenation. She has been an Adjunct Associate Professor at Touro College of Osteopathic Medicine since 2007 where she is involved in lecturing and teaching medical students in The Osteopathic Manipulative Medicine Department. Doctor Barbara is happily married and has five sons.

Doctor Barbara continues to always grow in medicine both in her medical skills and in educating both students and the public.

www.DoctorBarbara.com